Health, Drugs and Healing in C

T0227661

This volume contains five chapters written by American, European and Central Asian scholars, who examine a range of issues critical to our understanding of health and healing in contemporary Central Asia. Grounded in the review of medical literature in Arabic, Persian and Chaghatay Turkic, extensive field work in the Central Asian republics, and the examination of state and Communist Party archival records, this book offers a range of insights and new perspectives on this area.

The chapters of this edited volume survey largely unstudied medical texts produced and circulated in Central Asia from the sixteenth to twentieth centuries, provide a detailed account of the administrative regulation of addiction and Stalinist repression of opium users in Soviet Badakhshan, explore the complex relationships between biomedicine and indigenous healing practices and discourses, and discuss the politics and epidemiology of HIV/AIDS in Central Asia.

This book was published as a special issue of *Central Asian Survey.*

Alisher Latypov works as an international consultant on HIV, health and development issues. He completed his doctoral studies at the Wellcome Trust Centre for the History of Medicine at UCL, UK. Dr. Latypov is a member of the editorial boards of the International Journal of Drug Policy and Harm Reduction Journal.

Thirdworlds

Edited by Shahid Qadir, *University of London*

THIRDWORLDS will focus on the political economy, development and cultures of those parts of the world that have experienced the most political, social, and economic upheaval, and which have faced the greatest challenges of the postcolonial world under globalisation: poverty, displacement and diaspora, environmental degradation, human and civil rights abuses, war, hunger, and disease. **THIRDWORLDS** serves as a signifier of oppositional emerging economies and cultures ranging from Africa, Asia, Latin America, Middle East, and even those 'Souths' within a larger perceived North, such as the U.S. South and Mediterranean Europe. The study of these otherwise disparate and discontinuous areas, known collectively as the Global South, demonstrates that as globalisation pervades the planet, the south, as a synonym for subalterity, also transcends geographical and ideological frontiers.

Terrorism and the Politics of Naming
Edited by Michael Bhatia

Reconstructing Post-Saddam Iraq
Edited by Sultan Barakat

From Nation-Building to State-Building
Edited by Mark T. Berger

Connecting Cultures
Edited by Emma Bainbridge

The Politics of Rights
Dilemmas for feminist praxis
Edited by Andrea Cornwall and Maxine Molyneux

The Long War – Insurgency, Counter-insurgency and Collapsing States
Edited by Mark T. Berger and Douglas A. Borer

Market-led Agrarian Reform
Edited by Saturnino M. Borras, Jr.

After the Third World?
Edited by Mark T. Berger

Developmental and Cultural Nationalisms
Edited by Radhika Desai

Globalisation and Migration
New issues, new politics
Edited by Ronaldo Munck

Domestic and International Perspectives on Kyrgyzstan's 'Tulip Revolution'
Motives, mobilizations and meanings
Edited by Sarah Cummings

War and Revolution in the Caucasus
Georgia Ablaze
Edited by Stephen F. Jones

War, Peace and Progress in the 21st Century Development, Violence and Insecurities
Edited by Mark T. Berger and Heloise Weber

Renewing International Labour Studies
Edited by Marcus Taylor

Youth in the Former Soviet South Everyday Lives between Experimentation and Regulation
Edited by Stefan B. Kirmse

Political Civility in the Middle East
Edited by Frédéric Volpi

The Transformation of Tajikistan Sources of Statehood
Edited by John Heathershaw

Movement, Power and Place in Central Asia and Beyond Contested Trajectories
Edited by Madeleine Reeves

People Power in an Era of Global Crisis Rebellion, Resistance and Liberation
Edited by Barry K. Gills and Kevin Gray

EU Strategies on Governance Reform Between Development and State-building
Edited by Wil Hout

Identity, Inequity and Inequality in India and China Governing Difference
Edited by Ravinder Kaur and Ayo Wahlberg

The Personal and the Professional in Aid Work
Edited by Anne-Meike Fechter

Rising Powers and the Future of Global Governance
Edited by Kevin Gray and Craig N. Murphy

The Millennium Development Goals: Challenges, Prospects and Opportunities
Edited by Nana Poku

Development Perspectives from the Antipodes
Edited by Susanne Schech

Health, Drugs and Healing in Central Asia
Edited by Alisher Latypov

Health, Drugs and Healing in Central Asia

Edited by
Alisher Latypov

Routledge
Taylor & Francis Group
LONDON AND NEW YORK

First published 2014 by Routledge

Published 2014 by Routledge
2 Park Square, Milton Park, Abingdon, Oxfordshire OX14 4RN

and by Routledge
711 Third Avenue, New York, NY 10017

Routledge is an imprint of the Taylor and Francis Group, an informa business

First issued in paperback 2015

British Library Cataloguing in Publication Data
A catalogue record for this book is available from the British Library

ISBN 978-0-415-73911-5 (hbk)
ISBN 978-1-138-95472-4 (pbk)

Typeset in Times New Roman
by Taylor & Francis Books

Publisher's Note
The publisher accepts responsibility for any inconsistencies that may have arisen during the conversion of this book from journal articles to book chapters, namely the possible inclusion of journal terminology.

Contents

Citation Information

The chapters in this book were originally published in *Central Asian Survey*, volume 32, issue 1 (March 2013). When citing this material, please use the original page numbering for each article, as follows:

Chapter 1
Muslim medical culture in modern Central Asia: a brief note on manuscript sources from the sixteenth to twentieth centuries
Devin DeWeese
Central Asian Survey, volume 32, issue 1 (March 2013) pp. 3-18

Chapter 2
The opium war at the 'roof of the world': the 'elimination' of addiction in Soviet Badakhshan
Alisher Latypov
Central Asian Survey, volume 32, issue 1 (March 2013) pp. 19-36

Chapter 3
Mentally ill or chosen by spirits? 'Shamanic illness' and the revival of Kazakh traditional medicine in post-Soviet Kazakhstan
Danuta Penkala-Gawęcka
Central Asian Survey, volume 32, issue 1 (March 2013) pp. 37-51

Chapter 4
Prohibition, stigma and violence against men who have sex with men: effects on HIV in Central Asia
Alisher Latypov, Tim Rhodes and Lucy Reynolds
Central Asian Survey, volume 32, issue 1 (March 2013) pp. 52-65

Chapter 5
Kyrgyzstan: still a regional 'pioneer' in HIV/AIDS or living on its reputation?
Svetlana Ancker, Bernd Rechel, Martin McKee and Neil Spicer
Central Asian Survey, volume 32, issue 1 (March 2013) pp. 65-84

Please direct any queries you may have about the citations to clsuk.permissions@cengage.com

Notes on Contributors

Svetlana Ancker, Department of Health Services Research and Policy, London School of Hygiene & Tropical Medicine, London, UK

Devin DeWeese, Department of Central Eurasian Studies, Indiana University Bloomington, USA

Alisher Latypov, The Central Asia Program, Institute for European, Russian, and Eurasian Studies, The Elliott School of International Affairs, George Washington University, Washington DC, USA and Global Health Research Center of Central Asia (GHRCCA), Columbia University, New York, NY, USA

Martin McKee, Department of Health Services Research and Policy, London School of Hygiene & Tropical Medicine, London, UK

Danuta Penkala-Gawęcka, Department of Ethnology and Cultural Anthropology, Adam Mickiewicz University, Pozna⊠, Poland

Bernd Rechel, Department of Health Services Research and Policy, London School of Hygiene & Tropical Medicine, London, UK

Lucy Reynolds, London School of Hygiene and Tropical Medicine, London, UK

Tim Rhodes, London School of Hygiene and Tropical Medicine, London, UK

Neil Spicer, Faculty of Public Health and Policy, Department of Global Health and Development, London School of Hygiene & Tropical Medicine, London, UK

OBITUARY

Marie Bennigsen-Broxup (1944–2012)

Laurence Broers

Conciliation Resources, London, UK

It is with great regret that we announce the loss of Marie Bennigsen, an esteemed and valuable founding member of our community, on 7 December 2012. Marie took over the editorship of *Central Asian Survey* in 1987, the only scholarly journal of its era dedicated to Central Asia. She defined its remit broadly to provide a forum for the study not only of the five Central Asian republics, but also the broad swathe of predominantly Muslim Irano-Turkic peoples reaching from Anatolia to western China, including Soviet Muslim minorities. She also ensured that the journal featured articles about the Caucasus (never considered part of Central Asia geographically or culturally) and commissioned occasional special issues devoted (sadly) to the various wars and insurgencies of the post-Soviet North and South Caucasus, thus achieving broad coverage of the Russian/Soviet imperial zone. Marie acted as editor of *CAS* for over 20 years and played a key role in providing a forum on these under-studied peripheries in Eurasia.

Marie was born in Paris in 1944, the daughter of Russian émigré and scholar of Islam, Alexandre Bennigsen. During her early married life she lived in Hong Kong and Moscow where she worked for the *Financial Times*, before returning to London in 1980. From a broader interest in the Muslim world, Marie's academic interests came to focus on the theme of Muslim resistance within the former Soviet Union. She joined the Society for Central Asian Studies based in Oxford in 1981 and in 1983 published *The Islamic Threat to the Soviet State*, co-authored with her father. The significance of this work lay in its focus on the Muslim minorities in the Soviet Union, from the myriad nationalities of the North Caucasus, through to the Muslim republics of Tatarstan and Bashkortostan in the Volga region and Central Asia. These nationalities' experience of incorporation into the Soviet state and their relationship to Soviet power was, at the time, little known outside a very small circle of academics and policy specialists. The Bennigsens' study suggested that restive Muslim nationalities could be the driving force behind a future challenge to the Soviet Union, a view attaining wide popularity among Sovietologists in the 1980s.

It was the North Caucasus that would come to dominate both Marie's academic interests and her work as an activist and advocate. It was in this region, and in Chechnya in particular, that her hypothesis that Muslim peripheries would mobilize to resist Russian domination was most clearly substantiated, in the form of the first (1994–6) and second (1999–2009) Chechen wars. These conflicts were marked by extraordinary levels of violence and destruction, and particularly during the lingering insurgency phase of the second war, appalling human-rights violations. Marie would devote much of her later life to informing the world about these events and to supporting non-governmental organizations (NGOs) engaged in humanitarian relief for the populations affected.

Marie Bennigsen first travelled to Chechnya and neighbouring Dagestan in 1992, just after the Soviet collapse and as Chechnya was orienting itself towards a future independent of Russia. She became a close associate of the Chechen leadership, engaging in international advocacy for their cause. Marie firmly believed the on-going crisis in Chechnya could only be understood in the context of two centuries of Russian conquest of the North Caucasus. She regarded the Russian presence in the North Caucasus as a colonial one, and foresaw the possibility of the Russian Federation's eventual disintegration as a result of continued violence and misrule in the region.

Marie played an important role in researching and popularizing Chechen perspectives on the conflict with Russia. In addition to articles on the topic in *Central Asian Survey*, in 1992 she edited and contributed to *The North Caucasus barrier. The Russian advance towards the Muslim world*, a collection of articles premised on the notion that the North Caucasus had, in fact, been at war with Russia almost without interruption since the end of the eighteenth century. In 1998–9 Marie conducted interviews with 20 Chechen field commanders and staff officers, including Aslan Maskhadov, architect of the Chechen victory in the first Chechen war, subsequently elected president of the republic in 1997 and assassinated by Russian special forces in 2005.

Marie Bennigsen was a resolute non-conformist and her career consistently crossed boundaries between academia and rights activism. Those who worked with her attest to her readiness to challenge any authority and her generosity of spirit. She devoted considerable time and energy to charitable causes such as the Children of Chechnya Action Relief Mission, which supported the presence of a permanent hospital in the area of Georgia neighbouring Chechnya, implementing an anti-tuberculosis programme and treating Chechens displaced from the war-ravaged republic, as well as *ad hoc* medical missions to Chechnya itself through the 2000s. All those who knew her also attest to the fact that the Bennigsen-Broxup family home was for over three decades a frequent refuge for Chechens and other North Caucasians in Western Europe.

Marie's last project was the establishment of a new scholarly journal, *Caucasus Survey*, dedicated to the Caucasus. She remained convinced, to the last, of the need to pay more attention to local processes and perceptions in this volatile region rather than relying on grand geopolitical visions. She was in the process of establishing the journal when she died after a short illness; it is hoped that the project will be taken up by others.

Marie Bennigsen is survived by her husband, Michael Broxup, and their two sons.

Muslim medical culture in modern Central Asia: a brief note on manuscript sources from the sixteenth to twentieth centuries

Devin DeWeese

Department of Central Eurasian Studies, Indiana University Bloomington, USA

This article surveys the body of medical literature, in Arabic, Persian and Turkic, produced and circulated in Central Asia from the sixteenth to twentieth centuries, on the basis of catalogues of Islamic manuscript collections in the region, highlighting royal patronage of medical knowledge as well as the continuation of traditional modes of transmitting medical lore into the colonial and Soviet periods. The survey is a reminder that indigenous medical lore in Central Asia left a substantial body of still-unexplored sources, and that the encounter of traditional Central Asian medical practices with 'modern' medicine cannot reasonably be studied solely on the basis of Russian colonial or Soviet perspectives.

Traditional notions of health and disease in Central Asia are rooted in multiple worldviews and cultural conditionings that reflect various historical experiences, ranging from pre-Islamic times to the Soviet era. There can be no doubt, however, that throughout the region, and for a time-span ranging from 1200 years to a minimum of 300 years, the engagement of the peoples of Central Asia with Islam, in cultural, intellectual and religious terms, has determined the essential framework for understanding and managing health and illness. This is clear from indigenous Central Asian medical literature (which is steeped in the longstanding Muslim adaptation of Greek and Indian medical lore); it is clear from the range of accepted etiologies of illness (whether imbalances of humors, possessions, malicious 'magic' or other problems); it is clear from the basic history of medical culture in the region; and it is clear from the very vocabulary of health, illness and healing in the languages of all the region's contemporary peoples.

However, the domination of Central Asian studies by approaches rooted in Russian colonial, Soviet and Sovietological scholarly habits has obscured the pervasiveness of the Muslim cultural framework that has shaped Central Asian medical lore for more than a millennium, chiefly in two ways. First, such scholarship has been unable to draw upon familiarity with the historical medical traditions of Islamic civilization, or with the body of comparative material on the understanding of health and illness in the wider Muslim world. It has thus failed to recognize the inherently pluralistic character of Muslim medical lore, historically and at present, and its

---

Note: This survey is a byproduct of a paper prepared for a conference on 'Healing Paradigms and the Politics of Health in Central Asia', organized at Columbia University by the Global Health Research Center of Central Asia, in April 2011; my participation in the conference resulted not from any expertise on the history of medicine or health issues in Central Asia – I have none – but from my work as a student of religious life in the region, in recognition of the substantial impact of religion, broadly understood, upon notions of illness and health. The original paper included observations on two areas of overlap between religious activity and healing paradigms (shrine-centered religious practices focused on the restoration or maintenance of health and Sufi rites adapted as healing ceremonies), as well as the survey of Central Asian sources on medical history that is presented here.

accommodation of a wide range of practices, and practitioners, that were diverse in their origins, and remained diverse in their use (including modern Western medicine), but were all nevertheless 'processed' in a fully Muslim framework. Such scholarship has thus been susceptible to pseudo-historical constructions that divide indigenous Central Asian medical traditions into 'pre-Islamic' and 'Islamic' components,[1] or posit simple dichotomies, such as 'Muslim' vs. 'Western', 'traditional' vs. 'modern', or 'religious' vs. 'scientific', that are mostly unhelpful in understanding actual historical development, or in understanding actual contemporary life.

Second, in failing to understand the diversity of medical practices and paradigms in Central Asia as part of that region's participation in Muslim tradition, scholarship on Central Asia that is uninformed by the skills and analytical frameworks of Islamic studies has encouraged a neglect of the indigenous sources on medical history and the lore of health and illness. There has thus been little serious investigation into the prevailing medical cultures of Islamic Central Asia, on the eve of the Russian conquest or of the later establishment of Soviet power, or into the continuation of those 'pre-modern' medical cultures through the Tsarist and Soviet periods.[2]

The present brief survey is intended to offer some idea of the body of sources that might be usefully explored for a more historically grounded understanding of medical practices and notions of health and illness in Central Asia before the introduction of Western medicine. It gives an outline of the body of medical literature, in Arabic, Persian and Chaghatay Turkic, produced, circulated and 'consumed' in the Western parts of Central Asia from the sixteenth through the early twentieth century, chiefly on the basis of published catalogues representing the production and circulation of manuscripts in the region itself. It reflects not merely the ongoing copying of works comprising the shared inheritance of the classics of Islamic medical literature, but indigenous adaptations, translations and observationally augmented elaborations of such works, as well as original compilations intended for actual use and consultation by practising physicians. It is in no way exhaustive, and is presented without pretense of actually having begun to explore this rich medical corpus (a task best left to others). The extent of that body of sources should remind us, in turn, that the historical dimensions of the encounter between indigenous medical traditions and those brought to the region in the wake of the Russian conquest will only be properly assessed when the skills needed to utilize 'Islamic' manuscripts become a standard component of the training of those claiming an interest in Central Asian studies.

Central Asian Islamic medical literature remains overwhelmingly in manuscript form, and is preserved chiefly in Central Asian manuscript collections (above all in Tashkent);[3] it remains largely unstudied, but as a rule the more recent the work, the more likely it is to be found only in Central Asian collections (or in the former imperial capital, St Petersburg), and to have attracted minimal scholarly attention.[4] Even Central Asian scholars have tended to focus on earlier medical texts, such as the enormously influential *Qānūn* of the Bukharan-born Ibn Sīnā, a source of pride as a 'native son', rather than on works produced in more recent times. Ironically, the older 'classical' works are thus more familiar than works compiled in the sixteenth century or later, and interest in establishing the original text of the older works has naturally privileged the earliest manuscripts, rather than more recent copies that may include extensive comments and annotations reflecting comparison with other works or the results of actual experience.

In part the preference for the 'classical' works reflects a general pattern with Central Asian texts, but it also stems from the fact that Central Asian medical literature produced down through the thirteenth and fourteenth centuries is part of the larger Islamic medical tradition reflected in manuscript collections throughout the world, and studied as part of the larger whole.[5] Beginning with the Timurid era of the fifteenth century, however, Central Asian works build upon that Islamic medical tradition, but tend to become more isolated in their circulation, and increasingly reflect local developments that ought to be of prime interest for the history of medical concepts and practices in the region, but remain essentially unknown. Some Timurid-era works are found in manuscript collections outside Central Asia, to be sure, but they also remained influential in the region itself, as evidenced both in their ongoing use and elaboration by later Central Asian authors,[6] and in their continued copying, often with royal patronage.[7] A common trajectory sees such works copied and edited, for instance, through royal patronage in Ashtarkhānid times, and copied again under the patronage of the Manghït dynasty of nineteenth-century Bukhārā; 'copying' in each period was often accompanied by expansion, adaptation or annotation, thus rendering each 'copy' a distinctive window on the development of medical concepts and practices.

Both the isolation, and the 'local' copying and elaboration, increase with the advent of the Uzbek era in the sixteenth century, which saw substantial royal patronage of medical literature. The Shïbānid or Abū'l-Khayrid courts of Mawarannahr sponsored a number of influential medical works, beginning with the Persian *Dastūr al-'ilāj*, by Sulṭān 'Alī, known as 'Ṭabīb-i Khurāsānī', who served at the court of the *khān* Köchkünjī (r. 1510–30) in Samarqand and compiled this work in 933/1526. The work's composition was in fact proposed to him somewhat earlier by Maḥmūd Shāh Sulṭān, ruler of Akhsī (that is, Akhsīkat or Akhsīkent, in the Farghāna Valley), who summoned Sulṭān 'Alī to his court during an illness.[8] The *Dastūr al-'ilāj* did become known outside Central Asia,[9] as did a slightly later work written by Sulṭān 'Alī as a supplement or companion to the *Dastūr*, known as the *Muqaddima* ('introduction') to the *Dastūr al-'ilāj*, and dedicated to Abū Sa'īd b. Köchkünjī (r. 1530–3). This later work appears to have been widely distributed in the region, and surviving copies were sponsored by Ashtarkhānid and Manghït rulers.[10] At the beginning of the *Dastūr al-'ilāj*, the author affirms that he had worked as a physician for '40 years', gaining a reputation in Khurāsān and Mawarannahr, prior to his summons to Akhsī; in his *Muqaddima*, he refers to having served Köchkünjī's son Abū Sa'īd for 20 years prior to that later work's composition, suggesting his attachment to the court of Samarqand during much of the reign of Köchkünji. Sulṭān 'Alī's *Muqaddima* was translated into Chaghatay Turkic in Eastern Turkistan, in the eighteenth or nineteenth century.[11] As for the original *Dastūr al-'ilāj*, it was often copied locally, with some copies reflecting the work's ongoing use and 'adjustment' in various parts of Central Asia;[12] there is evidence, for instance, of the work's circulation in the Qazaq steppe during the early eighteenth century.[13]

Other medical works produced in the sixteenth century with local Central Asian patronage are known only from Central Asian manuscript collections. At the Köchkünjid court of Samarqand, another sixteenth-century author, Mullā Muḥammad Yūsuf-i Kaḥḥāl ('the eye-doctor'), served as the personal physician of 'Abd al-Laṭīf Khān b. Köchkünjī (who ruled as *khān* from 947–59/1540–51). His three known medical works are preserved together in a single manuscript, evidently copied in the seventeenth century, thus suggesting that they were not circulated as widely, or as recently, as the works of Sulṭān 'Alī. Mullā Muḥammad Yūsuf's *Taḥqīq al-ḥummayāt* (on fevers) was dedicated to 'Abd al-Laṭīf Khān,[14] while his *Risāla dar taḥqīq-i nabż va tafsīra* (on the pulse), was dedicated to Sulṭān Sa'īd Khān (a grandson of Köchkünjī, r. 975–80/1567–72);[15] both works refer to the author's teacher in medicine, 'Imād al-Dīn Mas'ūd, known as Mawlānā Mīr-kalān. Another of his works, the brief *Zubdat al-kaḥḥālīn*, on diseases of the eyes, was dedicated to a certain Mu'izz al-Dawla Khwāja Pāyanda Muḥammad.[16]

In 948/1541, also for 'Abd al-Laṭīf Khān, and thus no doubt in Samarqand, a certain Muḥammad Ḥusayn b. al-Mīrakī al-Samarqandī completed a copy of a Persian pharmacological work (the *Ikhtiyārāt-i Badī'ī*, written in 770/1369 by the court physician of the Muẓaffarids of Shīrāz, 'Alī b. Ḥusayn al-Anṣārī, known as Khwāja Zayn al-'Aṭṭār [d. 807/1404]); he added in the margins of the manuscript nearly 600 drawings of medicinal plants, animals, vessels for the preparation and preservation of medicines, and other sorts of illustrations,[17] reminding us of the potential value and 'originality' of later 'copies' of famous works.

At another Abū'l-Khayrid court, finally, in Tashkent, the physician Shāh 'Alī b. Sulaymān al-Kaḥḥāl produced the *Tadhkirat al-kaḥḥālīn*, completed in 951/1544–5, under Nawrūz Aḥmad Khān; it was a Persian adaptation and expansion of an Arabic work by the famous tenth-century physician of Baghdād, of Christian origin, 'Alī b. 'Īsā al-Kaḥḥāl.[18] A slightly later and more general work, the *Shifā' al-'alīl*, was written by 'Ubaydullāh b. Yūsuf 'Alī *al-kaḥḥāl*, between 970/1562–3 and 975/1567–8, and was dedicated to a son of Nawrūz Aḥmad, Muḥammad Darvīsh Bahādur Khān (i.e., the brother of Bābā Sulṭān, installed as ruler in Tashkent by the latter's enemy 'Abdullāh b. Iskandar).[19] The work covers ailments of individual organs 'from head to foot', as well as the preparation of medicines, and was based, the author writes, upon various classical medical works, as well as his own practical experience and that of his father, teachers and brothers, all of whom were renowned physicians of the age.

Though its authorship and patronage context remain unclear, another Persian work devoted to diseases of the eyes may be related to the court of 'Abdullāh b. Iskandar in Bukhārā. This is the *Żiyā-yi 'uyūn*, written in 978/1570; it consists of four chapters and a long conclusion that amounts to a glossary of medicinal substances. The work survives in a single known manuscript copied, in the year the work was completed, by a certain 'Arab-Muḥammad al-Bukhārī.[20]

The extensive royal patronage of Central Asian medical literature during the sixteenth century attests to the high importance placed on medical learning by a succession of *khāns*; this pattern of patronage evidently turned to active participation by rulers in the cultivation of medical knowledge during the seventeenth century. In Khwārazm, the famous *khān* Abū'l-Ghāzī (r. 1643–63), best known for his two Chaghatay Turkic historical works, is also ascribed the authorship of a Chaghatay medical work, entitled *Manāfi' al-insān*, preserved in a single manuscript copied in the first half of the nineteenth century.[21] That work, cited as Abū'l-Ghāzī's, was evidently utilized (along with the *Qānūn* of Ibn Sīnā and other works) in the composion of the Turkic *Multaqaṭ al-ṭibb*, evidently an original compilation rather than a translation; it was produced in Khwārazm by Ja'far Khwāja b. Naṣr al-Dīn Khwāja al-Ḥusaynī, of Hazārasp, in 1239/1823–4.[22] Several other Chaghatay medical works were written in Khwārazm in the era of the Qonghrat dynasty, in the nineteenth century, including a Turkic translation of a celebrated Arabic work from the twelfth century, the famous *Dhakhīra-yi Khwārazmshāhī*, by Zayn al-Dīn Ismā'īl Jurjānī.[23] Other late Chaghatay medical works, possibly of Khwārazmian provenance, are represented in single manuscripts, such as the anonymous *Risāla-yi shifā' al-abdān*, copied in 1271/1854.[24] More clearly of Khwārazmian provenance, but reflecting the period after the Russian conquest, is a Chaghatay translation of the Persian *Jāmi' al-favā'id*, known also as the *Ṭibb-i Yūsufī*, by the famous sixteenth-century physician Yūsuf b. Muḥammad b. Yūsuf Haravī, who lived under Bābur and Humāyūn; the translation was done in 1299/1882 by Mullā Muḥammad Amīn b. Mullā Muḥammad Ẓāhir Khwāja al-Ḥusaynī al-Khwārazmī, with the *takhalluṣ* 'al-Khādim', and survives in the translator's autograph.[25]

In Bukhārā and Balkh, meanwhile, several Ashtarkhānid rulers are known as sponsors of medical works.[26] An interesting treatise of a type belonging to the fringes of medical literature was prepared for Nadhr Muḥammad Khān, evidently during his time in Balkh, by a certain Qāżī Ḥāfiẓ Tūlak Andigānī (d. 1048/1638). The work, called simply his *risāla*, deals with the harmfulness of smoking tobacco and opium, and on the use of other substances (including nutmeg) regarded as prohibited; the author mostly cites works of jurists and theologians, but evidently describes the medical consequences of these drugs' use.[27] Subḥān Qulī Khān (r. 1681–1702) was especially interested in medical knowledge; among the products of his patronage are two late-seventeenth-century copies of Jurjānī's *Dhakhīra-yi Khwārazmshāhī*,[28] and he was also no doubt involved in the preparation of a copy of an anonymous seventeenth-century work on medicinal liquids (it bears the seal of Subḥān Qulī Khān's son, Muḥammad Muqīm Sulṭān, evidently reflecting a time prior to his independent rule in Balkh).[29]

Subḥān Qulī Khān, moreover, was evidently himself the author of a Persian medical work, entitled *Iḥyā' al-ṭibb-i Subḥānī*, which survives, as in the pattern noted earlier, in copies sponsored by Bukharan rulers of the Manghït dynasty in the nineteenth century.[30] The same *khān* is also ascribed authorship of an untitled Chaghatay work on medicine, preserved in a late manuscript in the collection of the Hungarian Academy of Sciences; it remains unclear whether and how this Turkic work is related to the Persian treatise ascribed to the *khān*.[31]

Also of special interest is a Chaghatay translation, evidently from Arabic, of a medical compilation entitled *Khulāṣat al-ḥukamā*; the translation was apparently done for (though in one copy, it is said to have been done *by*) the last Ashtarkhānid ruler, Abū'l-Fayż Khān (r. 1711–47), and survives in several manuscripts.[32] Though common in Khwārazm, especially in the nineteenth century, translations into Chaghatay (like Turkic literary production more generally) appear to have been quite rare in Bukhārā, lending this work significance from the standpoint of literary and linguistic, and not only medical, history.

The seventeenth, eighteenth and nineteenth centuries also saw the strong representation in Central Asia of medical works produced under Moghul patronage in India,[33] and, somewhat less prominently, under Ṣafavid patronage in Iran;[34] works reflecting Durrānī patronage from Afghanistan likewise circulated in the Manghït realm during the nineteenth century,[35] and some European works also began to appear in Central Asia in that period.[36] However, manuscript collections in Central Asia make it clear that royal patronage of the production and transmission of medical literature of 'local' origin continued throughout these centuries, leaving no doubt that the intellectual and 'scientific' stagnation typically ascribed to the region during this era (or during parts of it) did not apply to medical literature. Indeed, indigenous medical and pharmacological production by no means ended with the emergence of the 'tribal' dynasties that dominated Central Asia on the eve of the Russian conquest of the second half of the nineteenth century. Some works produced in Khwārazm under the Qonghrat dynasty were noted above; and even the independent ruler of Marv, a region not taken by the Manghïts of Bukhārā until 1785, appears to have patronized medical literature. A certain Sayyid Muḥammad, known by the poetic *takhalluṣ* 'Ḥasrat', wrote a substantial verse work, in Persian, describing the preparation of medicines, completing it in 1188/1774 and dedicating the first and second sections of the work (all that survives) to Bayrām-'Alī Khān, ruler of Marv, and his son Ḥusayn, respectively. The work is preserved in a unique manuscript, copied in 1261/1844–5 by Ḥājjī Muḥammad Samarqandī (and thus perhaps reflecting, at this stage, Bukharan patronage).[37]

In Bukhārā itself, Manghït patronage was especially strong during the reigns of Shāh Murād (1785–1800), Amīr Ḥaydar (1800–25) and Naṣrullāh (1827–60). One of the most interesting, and prolific, medical authors of Central Asia during this era enjoyed the patronage of Shāh Murād. This was Ṣāliḥ b. Muḥammad b. Muḥammad Ṣāliḥ Qandahārī Qā'inī, a native of the region of Herat who evidently began his medical writing before he came to the Manghït court. Perhaps his best-known work is a large pharmacopia entitled simply *'Amal-i Ṣāliḥ*, or *'Amal al-ṣāliḥīn*, which was evidently completed in 1180/1766–7, describing in detail the preparation of medicinal substances. In his introduction he declares that physicians should themselves study medicines rather than leaving their preparation to sellers of drugs and perfumes (that is, to *'aṭṭārs*), and affirms that he had studied the subject himself and had prepared a dictionary of medicines, with accounts of their preparation and proper dosing. At least four copies of this compilation survive,[38] as do two copies of a later work of the same type, the *Tuḥfat al-ṣāliḥīn*, finished in 1199/1785, evidently reflecting his move to Shāh Murād's court. One copy of the later work, which is organized into an introduction and 28 chapters (signaling an alphabetical arrangement), was owned by a later member of the Manghït dynasty.[39]

The same author also wrote two works on the diseases of children. One, entitled *Tuḥfa-yi shāyista*, was evidently completed in 1189/1775 (again, prior to his establishment at Shāh Murād's court). The introduction to the work discusses the impact of natural and environmental conditions on the child, and the rest of the work is divided into two parts, the first on illnesses affecting children from birth to age six, the second on older children, up to maturity.[40] The other, evidently later, is entitled *Tuḥfat al-ma'ṣūmīn*, and is known from two surviving manuscripts;[41] the author writes in the introduction that medical works known to him dealt with childhood illnesses inadequately or not at all, and insists that the majority of sick children could be saved from death if they were accorded proper medical care. He further discusses the importance of water, air and shelter for children's health, the necessity of cleanliness in preparing meals, and so on. The remainder of the work is divided into two sections (*maqāla*), the first dealing with infertility, pregnancy, illnesses of pregnant women and breastfeeding, and the second discussing children's diseases. The conclusion includes a section noting the importance of protecting children from drying winds, snakes and scorpions.

A focus on pediatrics is evidenced also in an anonymous fragment of a Persian medical work of likely Manghït patronage, bearing the heading *faṣl dar bayān-i bīmārī-yi gūdakān va mu'āl-lajāt* ('Section describing the illnesses of children and their treatment') preserved in a nineteenth-century manuscript.[42] A different concern is reflected in another work that may date from Shāh Murād's reign, namely the anonymous *Tadāruk al-sumūm*, in Persian, on the preparation of poisons; the work, structured in three sections (on poisons obtained from minerals, plants and animals), survives in a copy finished in 1215/1800.[43] Also of early nineteenth-century Bukharan provenance, it appears, is a substantial dictionary intended to explain medical terms in more commonly used words; it was compiled by a certain Muḥammad Ṣāliḥ al-Bukhārī, and was copied on Russian paper evidently in the early nineteenth century.[44] Amīr Ḥaydar's reign also saw the pattern of copying and expanding upon earlier works, noted above. This pattern continued under Amīr Naṣrullāh as well,[45] but original works were also produced in this era. A substantial commentary on the *Mīzān al-ṭibb*, a Persian medical work written in India under Awrangzīb, was completed in Bukhārā, in 1259/1843, by Muḥammad Sharīf b. Muḥammad Niyāz Bukhārī Naqshbandī, who dedicated his work to Naṣrullāh. From the author's introduction it appears that he worked on the commentary for nearly 15 years; it survives in a single copy.[46] Also under Naṣrullāh was produced a brief account of various medicinal substances, and the illnesses for which they were tried and found effective, compiled in 1255/1839 on the authority of two physicians, one called simply 'Mu'ālij-khān' and the other, his nephew, 'Ināyatullāh Kābulī.[47] A brief, anonymous medical 'handbook', entitled *Mukhliṣ al-mu'ālij* ('physician's friend'), was likewise compiled under Naṣrullāh, evidently, and survives in a copy from 1270/1853.[48] From this era as well, finally, survives a work of special interest, with regard to connections between Bukhārā and the Volga-Ural region, namely the collection of medical and pharmacological treatises (including a list of illnesses and their designations in Greek, Syriac, Arabic, Persian, Hindi and Türkī) copied in Bukhārā in the middle of the nineteenth century by one Muḥammad Ḥusayn al-Bulghārī *thumma* al-Bukhārī.[49]

A later member of the Manghït dynasty (one who never ruled), was clearly interested in the cultivation and preservation of medical knowledge reflected in such works. Sayyid Mīr Ṣiddīq, a son of Amīr Muẓaffar (whose reign, from 1860 until 1885, saw the khanate of Bukhārā transformed into a Russian protectorate), owned a sumptuous copy of Subḥān Qulī Khān's *Iḥyā'*, as mentioned above, and his seals appear also in an old copy of a more widely circulated fifteenth-century Persian medical work.[50] Mīr Ṣiddīq also owned a copy of an Arabic translation of the medical work of Paracelsus (see note 36), and a finely done copy of one of the works of

Ṣāliḥ Qā'inī Qandahārī (note 39). He himself was the copyist of a brief excerpt from a pharmacological work produced in India in the early eighteenth century.[51]

The production of indigenous medical literature continued after the Russian conquest of Central Asia. The second half of the nineteenth century and the first two decades of the twentieth yielded numerous anonymous works preserved in Central Asian manuscript collections, as well as, for example, a work on various foods (including breads and sweets) deemed medically useful, entitled *Kān-i ladhdhat va khwān-i ni'mat*, by Ibn Muḥammad 'Āshūr Raḥmatullāh al-Bukhārī, the famous Bukharan poet with the *takhalluṣ* 'Vāżiḥ' (d. 1311/1893–4).[52] From this era, also, date two works dealing with both moral and medical principles of sexual health, based on religious and medical sources. One, dealing with sexual relations and entitled simply *Risāla dar bāh*, was compiled by Qāżī Sayyid Qamar b. Qāżī Mīr Sayyid 'Ālim al-Ḥusaynī, *muftī* of Bukhārā for a time under Amīr Muẓaffar (r. 1860–85).[53] The other, entitled *Ṭiryāq-i istimnā*, describing the harmful effects of masturbation and methods for combating it, was written by Imām al-Dīn b. Shaykh Muḥammad 'Umar b. Shaykh Pīr Muḥammad, and survives in a single manuscript copied, in 1298/1880, by Amānullāh b. Akābir Khwāja Naqshband.[54]

A short compilation of medical lore, in both Chaghatay and Persian, was written by a certain Mullā Nūr Muḥammad, known as Mullā Yāmghūr-bāy, and copied by him, in 1320/1902, though in this case it is not certain where the manuscript was produced.[55] The same is true of an especially noteworthy production from this era, finally, namely the remarkable anonymous compilation, mostly in Persian but with extensive additions in Chaghatay, preserved in a unique manuscript copied in 1321/1903–4. The work, divided into 36 chapters, covers diseases and disorders of all parts of the body as well as directions for the preparation of medicines. As the account of the manuscript's contents makes clear, the work reflects a typical combination of detailed descriptions of various aspects of medical care and therapeutic practices with attention to religiously based cures or preventive measures (as, for instance, in the examples of various textual amulets used to prevent specific illnesses).[56] A similar, but smaller, compilation appears to date from the late nineteenth century, and is a kind of physician's handbook, with citations of classical authors, illustrations of vessels for preparing medicines, descriptions of diseases of specific organs and body parts, and so on. The anonymous author refers to a public health crisis he was sent to deal with in Nasaf, that is, Qarshī, in 1302/1885.[57]

The medical literature produced in nineteenth-century Khoqand under Ming rule was somewhat less extensive than the rich production in Bukhārā, but included some noteworthy works. None other than the poet Ḥādhiq, that is, Junaydullāh b. Shaykh al-Islām [*sic*], killed on order of Amīr Naṣrullāh in 1259/1843, wrote a commentary, entitled *Taḥqīq al-qavā'id*, on the *Qānūncha* of al-Chaghminī (d. 745/1344), itself a shortened version of Ibn Sīnā's *Qānūn*. Ḥādhiq's work was written in Khoqand in 1238/1822, under 'Umar Khān, at the request of the poet's friends.[58] Also evidently from the Farghāna Valley is an untitled Chaghatay medical work, surviving in three copies, based in part on the Persian *Jāmi' al-favā'id* of Yūsuf b. Muḥammad b. Yūsuf Yūsufī al-Haravī (written for Bābur in India, known as the *Ṭibb-i Yūsufī*). One copy, the earliest, was made by Dhākir Khwāja *ūrāq* b. Maḥmūd Khwāja Īshān Andigānī, for his personal use, in 1263/1846–7.[59]

Also in the Farghāna Valley, but already under Russian rule, the local scholar Maḥmūd Ḥakīm Yayfānī Khūqandī, born in 1851, compiled a substantial medical work entitled *Ṭarīq al-'ilāj*, in four sections (*maqāla*), of which only the third and fourth survive; the work was completed in 1910, and was lithographed in 1913. A manuscript containing part of the third *maqāla*, on anatomy (*tashrīḥ*) has also survived.[60] The same author evidently wrote another medical work, entitled *Qānūn al-'ilāj*, which has evidently not come down to us, as well as a brief Chaghatay historical work on the khanate of Khoqand, entitled *Khullaṣ al-tavārīkh*, completed in 1332/1913–14, which survives in two copies.[61]

The Persian work of Yūsufī noted above in connection with a Khoqandian adaptation, in effect, in Chaghatay was translated into Chaghatay by a nineteenth-century Khwārazmian author, as mentioned earlier. Yet another Chaghatay translation was produced in the Tsarist era by a remarkable scholar of Tashkent active in the late nineteenth and early twentieth centuries. This was Muḥammad Shāh Khwāja Tāshkandī, whose translation was done, he writes, for the benefit of the population of 'Turkistān', and was lithographed in Tashkent in 1316/1898, under the title *Tarjima-yi Shāhī.*[62] The same figure may be identified more fully as Muḥammad Shāh Khwāja Tāshkandī, the son of Shāh Fayżī Khwāja Shaykh-Khāvand-i Ṭahūrī (this *nisba* identifies him as a descendant of one of the 'patron saints' of Tashkent, the fourteenth-century Shaykh Khāvand-i Ṭahūr or 'Shaykh Antaur', whose shrine was a prominent site in the city-quarter of Tashkent that came to bear the saint's name). He was also responsible for a singular product of the early Soviet era, namely a unique manuscript preserving the Arabic text of Chaghminī's *Qānūncha* together with an interlinear Chaghatay translation; it is not clear when the translation was done, but the manuscript was copied in 1344/1925–6.[63]

Likewise in Tashkent, but later in the Soviet era, we know of two brothers active in the production and copying of Chaghatay medical works. The elder brother, Ḥāmid-khān (1870–1953), son of Muḥammad Ṣādiq-khān Shāshī, made the copy of Yayfānī's medical work noted above, and evidently made an abbreviation of one of his younger brother's medical works.[64] The younger brother, Bāsiṭ-khān (1878–1959), evidently wrote three large medical works that survive in manuscript form: (1) *Qānūn al-mabsūṭ*, also called *Qānūn-i Bāsiṭī*, based on Ibn Sīnā's *Qānūn* and commentaries upon it, completed in late November 1942, and surviving in a manuscript that runs to 310 folios;[65] (2) *Istilāḥāt al-aṭibbā fī intifā'āt al-aḥibbā*, a medical dictionary, giving Arabic terms and their 'Uzbek' equivalents or explanations, known also as the *Farhang al-mabsūṭ*, surviving in a manuscript completed in June 1944 and running to 136 folios; and (3) *Favā'id al-advīya va mavā'id al-aghdhīya*, a work on medicines, completed evidently in 1950, but intended as the first volume of a series of works that was ultimately left unfinished due to the author's failing health.[66]

The activity of these brothers should remind us, again, of the continuation of indigenous patterns of the production and transmission of medical lore, and of traditional manuscript culture more broadly, well into the Soviet era. It may also remind us that a fuller assessment of conceptions and traditions related to healing and illness cannot proceed on the assumption that the kind of medical lore reflected in Central Asian medical literature of the sixteenth to twentieth centuries, and 'internalized' more generally in both public and learned understandings of health and disease, was somehow swept away entirely by the changes of the Soviet era.

This brief survey is offered by way of showing that there is, in fact, a substantial body of sources reflecting the cumulative and often observationally based development of medical knowledge in Central Asia prior to the Russian conquest, and still later, outside the framework of Tsarist and Soviet policy. Many more examples could no doubt be offered through new work in the collections themselves; the present remarks are based solely on materials reflected in Russian-language manuscript catalogues produced in Soviet times,[67] which could have been utilized by earlier scholars interested in Central Asia in order to dispel the notion that understanding the encounter of indigenous medical traditions with those introduced through Russian or Soviet power could be achieved solely on the basis of Russian sources. It should be clear that our understanding of Central Asian medical lore (and, by extension, our constructions of the encounter of Russian and Western medical practices with indigenous traditions) cannot be said to have a serious foundation unless and until this literature is properly explored and assessed.

Notes

1. For a preliminary discussion of assumptions about 'pre-Islamic' vs. 'Islamic' origins in the ethnography of religion in Central Asia, see DeWeese (2011). Such assumptions appear not only in scholarship shaped by Soviet training, but also in Western studies shaped by the legacies of 'Sovietology'; see, with regard to notions of health and illness, the account of healing practices among the Qazaqs in Michaels (2003, 22, 24 ff.).
2. For a discussion of more balanced approaches to the social history of medicine in other parts of the Muslim world, see the review article of Gallagher (2012). The study of Central Asia, by contrast, remains plagued by two trends that promote the neglect of sources produced from the sixteenth to twentieth centuries. Sovietological works, uncritically admiring of 'modernity', do so from a later perspective, while scholarship focused on a presumed classical 'golden age' often does so from an earlier vantage point; for an extreme example of the latter, see the denunciations of 'modernity' in Beckwith (2009), where the historical development of Central Asia during the early-modern and modern eras is entirely ignored, and sources of the type outlined here are implicitly denied value.
3. The most important collection is that of the Institute of Oriental Studies of the Academy of Sciences of Uzbekistan (the 'Beruni institute'), in Tashkent; for its manuscripts, the basic guide remains the 11-volume *SVR*. The relevant volume of the catalogue of the major manuscript collection in Dushanbe (that of the Institute of Oriental Studies), *KVR*, was also consulted for the present survey.
4. For a brief overview of medical literature preserved in manuscript collections in Uzbekistan, see Shterenshis (2000). A more substantial survey of Islamic medical history with reference to manuscripts preserved in Tashkent is Hikmätulläev (1994), in which, alongside some brief studies and Uzbek translations of several Arabic medical works, the author gives a biographical survey of medical authors represented in the Tashkent collection (18–109). Uzbek translations of parts of many medical works, based on manuscripts preserved in Tashkent, are provided (with discussion of the works and their authors) in Häsäniy (1993).
5. For an overview of Muslim medical history and literature, see Savage-Smith (2000); for Arabic works of the classical period, see Sezgin (1970); for Persian medical literature, covering later works as well, see Storey (1971), and the older work (also covering Arabic sources) of Fonahn (1910). Hofman (1969) includes a brief section on authors of medical works in Chaghatay Turkic (VI, 241–9); like much of Hofman's coverage, this sketch was rendered obsolete by the absence of reference to the seventh volume of *SVR* (devoted exclusively to Turkic works, mostly in Chaghatay), which appeared already in 1964.
6. For example, an Arabic commentary on an early thirteenth-century medical work by Najīb al-Dīn Samarqandī (d. 619/1222), *Sharḥ al-asbāb va'l-'alāmāt*, by a native of Kirmān, Nafīs b. 'Avaż, who was invited by Ulugh Beg to Samarqand (the commentary was written there in 827/1424): MS Tashkent, 2872 (467 ff., ascribed to the seventeenth century; here and throughout the notes, the number given after 'MS Tashkent' is the manuscript's Inventory Number), *SVR*, I, 256, No. 568 (see Hikmätulläev [1994, 77–9]). This work did become known outside Central Asia, and is found in manuscript collections elsewhere; within Central Asia, it was admired and utilized by a medical author active in Marv in the 1770s (see below, note 37, and Häsäniy [1993, 114]), and was the chief basis for a compilative description of the symptoms of illnesses 'from head to foot' (a common genre in eighteenth- to nineteenth-century Central Asia), described at *SVR*, VIII, 103–4, No. 5686 (Inv. No. 8312/I, ff. 1a–53b, copied in 1233/1817), suggesting the ongoing elaboration of medical traditions. On the author of the original work, see Storey (1971, 215), and Levey and al-Khaledy (1967).
7. For example, Manṣūr b. Muḥammad b. Aḥmad, *Risāla dar tashrīḥ-i badan-i insān*, a work on anatomy dedicated to Tīmūr's grandson Pīr Muḥammad. The work is known from European manuscript collections, and was lithographed in the nineteenth century; at least one copy in Tashkent reflects Ashtarkhānid patronage: MS Tashkent, 2105 (57 ff., described in *SVR*, I, 255, No. 566; cf. Hikmätulläev [1994, 73]), copied, with notes and corrections, in 1101/1683, by a certain 'Arabshāh, who identifies himself only as a *banda-yi dargāh* ('servant of the court'), at the order of Subḥān Qulī Khān. The copyist also added six illustrations representing the skeleton, the nervous system, internal organs and so on. (The illustration of the skeleton, on f. 19b, is reproduced in the catalogue, facing p. 254). Another copy, MS Tashkent, 3663/V (ff. 331b–367a, *SVR*, IX, 283, No. 6436), copied in Kabul at the beginning of the nineteenth century, includes the illustration of the skeleton, as well as several pages left blank, presumably for further illustrations. Another Timurid-era medical work following a similar trajectory is a pharmacopia entitled *Baḥr al-khavāṣṣ*, dealing with the medicinal properties of various

substances; the apparently unique copy (see Storey [1971, 228]) indicates that the original work, completed in 867/1462–3 by Ni'matullāh al-Kirmānī, known as Ḥakīmī (who served for a time at the court of Sulṭān Ḥusayn Bāyqarā), was copied under Subḥān Qulī Khān, and was then compared with other medical works and corrected to produce the surviving copy, evidently prepared for Shāh Murād or Amīr Ḥaydar: MS Tashkent, 2146 (366 ff., *SVR*, I, 284, No. 642; however, Hikmätulläev [1994, 79–80], writes that this manuscript was copied for Subḥān Qulī Khān, without mention of the later stage in the manuscript's production). Some Timurid works, to be sure, had a shorter patronage sequence. An anonymous Persian medical work (called only *Risāla-yi Suhaylīya dar ṭibb*), evidently produced at the Timurid court of Herat, survives only in a copy made in the middle of the sixteenth century (MS Tashkent, 11,541, 218 ff.; *SVR*, X, 119–20, No. 6866, with the opening page shown on p. 121); another work, an Arabic medical dictionary, with descriptions of illnesses and medicines, entitled *Baḥr al-javāhir*, was evidently produced under Timurid patronage by Muḥammad b. Yūsuf of Herat, and is preserved outside Central Asia, but copies produced and preserved in Central Asia were likewise copied no later than the sixteenth century: MSS Tashkent, 2464 (419 ff., ascribed to the fifteenth century, *SVR*, I, 256, No. 567); 7192 (165 ff., copied 997/1589 in Kesh [Shahrisabz], *SVR*, V, 273–4, No. 3923).

8. This may refer to a grandson of the prominent Abū'l-Khayrid Jānī-bek; in the course of Muḥammad Shïbānī Khān's conquests, his uncle Jānī-bek was briefly allotted the region of Akhsī, but it is not clear whether this grandson, Maḥmūd b. Sulaymān b. Jānī-bek, ruled in the region. The description of the British Library's copy of the *Dastūr al-'ilāj* (Add. 17,947, in 230 ff., completed in 1060/1650), in Rieu (1881, II, 473), incorrectly renders Maḥmūd Shāh's seat of rule as 'Ajnī'.
9. See Storey (1971, 233–4, covering the *Dastūr al-'ilāj* and the *Muqaddima*). The work was lithographed several times in India in the late nineteenth century.
10. One Tashkent copy of the *Muqaddima-yi Dastūr al-'ilāj*, MS Tashkent, 2264/I, ff. 7b–97b (*SVR*, IX, 297–8, No. 6453), bears seals of 'Abd al-'Azīz Khān, dated 1071/1660–1, and of 'Abd al-'Azīz Khwāja b. Naṣr al-Dīn Khwāja al-Ḥusaynī, dated 1212/1797 and 1230/1814–15; another (10,925/VI, ff. 88a–151a, *SVR*, IX, 298, No. 6455) was copied in 1261/1845 by Nūr Muḥammad Khuttalānī; a third (7269/I, ff. 1b–94a, *SVR*, IX, p. 299, No. 6456) was produced already after the Russian conquest, in 1296/1879; and a fourth was copied in 1216/1801, but in Kabul (3663/II, ff. 15b–77b, *SVR*, IX, 298, No. 6454).
11. The *Muqaddima-yi Dastūr al-'ilāj* of Sulṭān 'Alī was rendered into Chaghatay by an unknown translator in Yarkand; one copy survives (MS Tashkent, 11,124, 140 ff., first half of the nineteenth century; *SVR*, VII, 293, No. 5449). It is briefly discussed in Hikmätulläev (1994, 81, 117–8), with a short excerpt from the introduction given in Cyrillic Uzbek transcription. An earlier medical work reflecting Chaghatayid patronage in Eastern Turkistan during the early sixteenth century is not represented in the collections of Tashkent or Dushanbe. This is the *Tuḥfa-yi khānī*, written by a certain Maḥmūd b. Muḥammad 'Abdullāh (who studied medicine in Shīrāz) and dedicated to Sulṭān Sa'īd Khān (r. 1514–33); see Storey (1971, 232–3).
12. Copies of the *Dastūr al-'ilāj* in Tashkent include Inv. Nos. 757 (240 ff., undated, copied by Bek-Muḥammad b. Sayyid Muḥammad), *SVR*, I, 264, No. 591; 2264/II (ff. 106a–366b, copied in 998/1589 by Bāqī Muḥammad b. Bābā Aḥmad Sāgharjī), *SVR*, I, 264, No. 592; 11,297 (282 ff., copied in 1281/1864–5 by Mullā Ḥusayn b. Mullā Qurbān, 'Ṭabīb-i Harātī'), *SVR*, IX, 296, No. 6451; 7269/II (ff. 94b–446a, copied in 1296/1879 by Ḥabībullāh b. 'Abd al-Sallām), *SVR*, IX, 297, No. 6452; and 3663/III (ff. 79b–326b, copied 1216/1801 by Mīrzā Ṣāliḥ Ḥakīm, a native of Lahore then dwelling in Kabul), *SVR*, IX, 296, No. 6450. See also the manuscripts in Dushanbe described in *KVR*, VI, Nos. 2228–2229 (both copied in the early nineteenth century). According to Hikmätulläev (1994, 80–2), the Tashkent collection holds seven copies of the *Dastūr al-'ilāj*; he adds that Inv. No. 2264 was owned by Sharīf-jān Makhdūm (d. 1932), a famous Bukharan *qāżī* and bibliophile (on whom see Allworth and Shukurov [2004], and Vokhidov and Choriev [2007]).
13. One Tashkent copy of the Persian *Dastūr al-'ilāj*, 11,261/I (ff. 1b–261b) [*SVR*, IX, 295–6, No. 6449], was completed in Rajab 1140/February 1728, evidently in the Chū Valley, upon the order of 'Khudāybanda Bahādur Ghāzī, known as (*mulaqqab be-*) Erke Khān b. 'Abd al-Rashīd', who must have been a Chinggisid ruling among the Qazaqs (note the manuscript's date, in the midst of the period of intense Junghar pressure on the Qazaqs of this region). The manuscript was later in the possession of a physician named 'Bāsiṭ Khān Zāhid Khān-oghlï', of 'old Tashkent' in Syrdar'inskaia oblast'; the same figure's seal also appears in a late nineteenth-century copy of the *Jāmi' al-favā'id* of Yūsuf b. Muḥammad b. Yūsuf al-Haravī, that is, the work known as *Ṭibb-i Yūsufī* (on which see below, notes 25, 33 and 62): Inv. No. 11,259 (83 ff., a nineteenth-century copy), *SVR*, IX, 294–5, No. 6448.

14. MS Tashkent, 2275/IX (ff. 179a–202b), *SVR*, IX, 304, No. 6469.
15. MS Tashkent, 2275/VI (ff. 108a–132b), *SVR*, IX, 309–10, No. 6475.
16. MS Tashkent, 2275/VIII (ff. 172a–178a), *SVR*, IX, 305, No. 6470; on the author and his works, see Hikmätulläev (1994, 86–7). The Khwāja Pāyanda Muḥammad mentioned as the patron of this work is perhaps to be identified with the Mawlānā Pāyanda Muḥammad whom ʻAbdullāh Khān b. Iskandar appointed to teach in his newly completed *madrasa* in Bukhārā in 974/1566–7 (see Ḥāfiẓ Tanïsh [1983, 259]), but Muḥammad Yūsuf's activity chiefly in Samarqand may render this identification less likely.
17. MS Tashkent, 1598, *SVR*, I, 282–3, No. 636 (281 ff.); for other copies of the work, evidently without illustrations (but including several from the sixteenth century), see *SVR*, I, 283–4, Nos. 637–41, and *SVR*, IX, 350–2, Nos. 6521–5 (according to Hikmätulläev [1994, 73–4], the Tashkent collection holds 20 copies of the work in all). On the *Ikhtiyārāt* and its author, see Storey (1971, 220–3).
18. One manuscript containing this Persian rendering, copied in 1225/1810, is preserved in Tashkent (Inv. No. 1832, *SVR*, I, 243–4, No. 545, noted in Storey [1971, 204]). Two other copies are preserved in Dushanbe: *KVR*, VI, 180-82, Nos. 2205 (ascribed to the late seventeenth century, in 137 ff.), and 2206 (an incomplete copy from the nineteenth century, evidently done by Mullā ʻAvaż Badal b. Mullā Muḥammad Sharīf Jūybārī). On other Persian adaptations of the work of ʻAlī b. ʻĪsā al-Kaḥḥāl, see Storey (1971, 203–5). Another work evidently by the same Shāh ʻAlī b. Sulaymān al-Kaḥḥāl is preserved in Tashkent, Inv. No. 4935/II (ff. 9b–41a, copied in 1008/1599 by a physician named Mawlānā ʻAbd al-ʻAzīz), *SVR*, IX, 286–7, No. 6439; however, the work is dated, in the catalogue (on the basis of a chronogram), to 905/1499–1500, suggesting a misreading, given the date of this author's other work.
19. Two surviving manuscripts of the *Shifā' al-ʻalīl* were copied in the same year, 1072/1662. The slightly older one, MS Tashkent, 2477/I, runs to 471 ff. (*SVR*, I, 271–2, No. 609, with a good description of the contents); evidently neither the copyist nor the place he worked is mentioned. The other copy from 1072/1662 is Inv. No. 2265, in 400 ff., copied in Balkh by Muslim b. Muḥammad al-Abīvardī (*SVR*, IX, 306–8, No. 6472), probably reflecting Ashtarkhanid patronage; this manuscript was bound in 1284/1867–8, and was purchased for 10,000 *tanga*s by Sharīf-jān Makhdūm (mentioned above, note 12), evidently in or after 1318/1900–1. Another essentially full copy of the work, MS Tashkent, 2611, in 393 ff., was evidently copied in the mid-nineteenth century (*SVR*, IX, 308–9, No. 6474), and bears the seal of an owner, a certain Mullā Mīr Ẓuhūr al-Dīn, dated 1298/1880–1. A fourth partial copy of the same work, completed in 1268/1852, contains only the section on childhood illnesses (Inv. No. 2629/II, ff. 396b–417b; *SVR*, IX, 308, No. 6473). The author, ʻUbaydullāh b. Yūsuf ʻAlī *al-kaḥḥāl*, and his work are briefly discussed in Hikmätulläev (1994, 84–5).
20. MS Tashkent, 10,299, 102 ff., copied in 978/1570 (*SVR*, X, 120, 122, No. 6867, with the first page shown on p. 123).
21. Abū'l-Ghāzī's *Manāfiʻ al-insān* is preserved in MS Tashkent, 4107 (64 ff., defective at the end, dated to the first half of the nineteenth century), described in *SVR* VII, 294, No. 5450; f. 2a of the manuscript is reproduced on p. 295 of the catalogue volume. The work is noted as Abū'l-Ghāzī's, with a brief excerpt from the introduction given in Cyrillic Uzbek, in Hikmätulläev (1994, 91–2).
22. MS Tashkent, 3336 (167 ff., copied 1243/1827–8, evidently an autograph), *SVR*, VII, 304, No. 5467; the work was dedicated to Sayyid Aḥmad al-Ḥusaynī, identified as 'a Khwārazmian shaykh'. According to Hikmätulläev (1994, 97–8), the author gives his own genealogy on ff. 165b–167a.
23. The Chaghatay translation of Jurjānī's *Dhakhīra-yi Khwārazmshāhī* survives in a single incomplete copy: MS Tashkent, 8263/I, ff. 1b–72b, *SVR* VII, 284, No. 5443 (the inventory number is given as 8203/I in Hikmätulläev [1994, 62]); the catalogue description assigns the manuscript to the eighteenth century, which if correct would make it clear that the translation preceded the extensive Khivan translation programme under the Qonghrats, in the mid-nineteenth century, but the dating seems unlikely. On Zayn al-Dīn Ismāʻīl Jurjānī (d. 531 or 535/1136–7 or 1140–1) and his work, see Storey (1971, 207–11). Several other late Chaghatay medical works are represented in single manuscripts, and some at least may be of Khwārazmian provenance; see *SVR*, VII, 301–3, Nos. 5460–5. Here too may be noted the Chaghatay translation of a Persian '*Risāla-yi ṣaydīya*', on the medical use of various animal parts (and on methods for hunting as indicated in the title), which appears to be of Khwārazmian provenance; see the introduction to Häsäniy and Yoldasheva (1994), where the editors note that a manuscript of the Persian original is preserved in Tashkent at the Institute of Oriental Studies, but give no Inventory No. for either the Persian or the Chaghatay manuscript.
24. MS Tashkent, 436/V (ff. 114b–128b, copied 1271/1854), *SVR* I, 280, No. 629.

25. MS Tashkent, 8391 (143 ff., dated 1299/1882), *SVR*, VII, 292, No. 5448; cf. Hikmätulläev (1994, 117), and Häsäniy (1993, 49, giving the Inv. No. as 8931).
26. From the early Ashtarkhanid era, a copy of a fourteenth-century Persian commentary on an abbreviated version of Ibn Sīnā's *Qānūn* was completed in 1016/1607 by Shaykh-zāda Muḥammad b. Shaykh-jān al-Karmīnī al-Bukhārī (MS Tashkent, 2492, *SVR*, I, 249, No. 551), but it is not entirely clear that the copy was prepared for a royal patron. A short excerpt from a work by a certain Muḥammad Ṣāliḥ b. Qutluq-biy, entitled simply *Risāla-yi ḥikmat* or *Risāla dar bayān-i mu'ālajāt-i ṭibbī*, is given in Uzbek translation in Häsäniy (1993, 253–5), with reference to a manuscript in Tashkent (Inv. No. 1810) copied in 1724; it is not clear where or when the work was written.
27. MS Tashkent, 2320, 58 ff., copied, evidently, before 1055/1645 (*SVR*, V, 351, No. 4054); cf. Inv. No. 2900/III, ff. 23b–31b (copied 1215/1800; *SVR*, V, 352, No. 4055), containing only the end of the work. See the discussion in Hikmätulläev (1994, 90–1).
28. MSS Tashkent, 433 (624 ff., dated 1108/1696), *SVR*, I, 251–2, No. 557; and 2111 (672 ff., dated 1109/1697), *SVR*, I, 252, No. 558.
29. MS Tashkent, 2275/I (ff. 1b–57a, evidently copied in the seventeenth century); *SVR*, IX, 365–6, No. 6540.
30. The *Iḥyā' al-ṭibb-i Subḥānī* survives in three complete copies in Tashkent: Inv. Nos. 2101 (301 ff., copied at the request of Amīr Ḥaydar, but not completed, evidently, until 1248/1832, by one 'Abdullāh Kātib), *SVR*, I, 265–6, No. 597; 3605/I (ff. 1b–135b, copied in 1212/1797 by Ūzbek Khwāja Mīr Ḥaydarī), *SVR*, IX, 319–20, No. 6485 (Hikmätulläev [1994, 94–5], mentions this manuscript alone when discussing the work); and 9750/II (ff. 4b–358b, copied 1249/1834 in Bukhārā by Ghulām Bahā' al-Dīn), *SVR*, IX, 320, No. 6486 (a partial copy of the work appears in Inv. No. 3605/II, ff. 137b–193b, dated to 1261/1845, *SVR*, IX, 321, No. 6487). Another incomplete copy, evidently made in 1257/1841, is held in Dushanbe (*KVR*, VI, 220–1, No. 2274 (Inv. No. 75/I, ff. 1b–51b), and what is likely a full copy, dated 1256/1840, is held in St Petersburg; see Miklukho-Maklai (1964, 36, No. 30). The first Tashkent copy noted here, Inv. No. 2101, bears seals indicating that it belonged to Sayyid Mīr Ṣiddīq, a son of the Manghït Amīr Muẓaffar (r. 1860–85).
31. The manuscript of the Turkic work was obtained in Herat by Vámbéry, who published portions of the text, with a German translation, in Vámbéry (1867, 164–72). See now the description of the work in László (2006; I am indebted to Ruth Meserve for a copy of this article); László does not mention the Persian work ascribed to Subḥān Qulī Khān, though he does cite Hofman, who mentions the Persian and Turkic works and affirms that the dispositions do not agree (Hofman [1969, VI, 245–6, and IV, 271]). No doubt direct examination of the Persian work will be required to determine the relationship, if any, between the two texts. In this connection, a Persian astrological work by the same *khān* is preserved in a nineteenth-century Khivan translation (MS Tashkent, 1205, 42 ff., copied 1272/1855–6, *SVR*, VII, 266–7, No. 5424), perhaps suggesting a similar trajectory for the *khān*'s medical work.
32. See *SVR*, VII, 297–9, Nos. 5451–6 (all evidently nineteenth-century copies), and a copy from 1277/1860 (*SVR* I, 280, No. 631, Inv. No. 436/III, ff. 66b–104b), ascribed to Ḥāfiẓ-i Kalān b. Badr al-Dīn Qārī, and not identified as a translation). A brief section from the latter manuscript is translated into Uzbek in Häsäniy (1993, 258–9, with the work described as the original work of Ḥāfiẓ-i Kalān from 1860 [see 390, note 238]).
33. For medical works of Moghul patronage, some preserved in copies of Indian origin brought to Central Asia, but some copied in Central Asia, see *SVR*, I, 266–7, Nos. 598–600 (evidently Indian copies), 268–70, Nos. 602–6 (at least one manuscript copied in Bukhārā), 272–4, Nos. 610–12 (evidently not Central Asian copies), 289–90, Nos. 655–6; *SVR*, IX, 312–15, Nos. 6479–80, 321–33, Nos. 6488–6501 (some Indian and some Central Asian copies), 356–61, Nos. 6533–6, 366–74, Nos. 6542–8 (No. 6533, a copy of a medical work compiled under Jahāngīr in 1036/1626–7, was copied in Bukhārā in 1279/1863 by Muḥammad Murād b. Mīrzā Qoldash, who copied many of the medical manuscripts in the Tashkent collection); *SVR*, V, 279, No. 3926 (an Indian copy); *SVR*, X, 114–19, Nos. 6861–5 (all but the first in a single seventeenth-century manuscript from India), and *KVR*, VI, 194-8, Nos. 2233–8 (most apparently produced in Central Asia), 216–17, Nos. 2267–8. On the circulation of Moghul medical works in Central Asia, see further Hikmätulläev (1994, 87–9, 92–4), Häsäniy (1993, 231–3), and the Uzbek translation of one such work, Häsäniy (1991), with excerpts also in Häsäniy (1993, 98–112). For various works by the celebrated 'Yūsufī', that is, Yūsuf b. Muḥammad b. Yūsuf Haravī, who lived under Bābur and Humāyūn, preserved in nineteenth-century Central Asian manuscripts, see *SVR*, I, 258–64, Nos. 572–590; *SVR*, IX, 291–5, Nos. 6441–8, 299–304, Nos. 6457–68 (mostly ninteenth-century Central Asian copies); see also *KVR*, VI, 182–91, Nos. 2207–27, 214, No. 2265 (on Yūsufī, see Storey [1971, 235–40]; Häsäniy

[1993, 47–50, 190–3, with translations from four of his works, 51–98, 193–206]; Hofman [1969, VI, 148–62]; and Shterenshis [2000, 101]).

34. For medical works of Safavid patronage, see *SVR*, I, 265, Nos. 594–6, and 270–1, Nos. 607–8; *SVR*, V, 276–9, Nos. 3929–35 (Indian and Central Asian copies); *SVR*, IX, 315–19, Nos. 6481–4 (some Indian, some Central Asian copies), 354–6, Nos. 6528–32, 361–2, No. 6537, 363–5, No. 6539; and *KVR*, VI, 192–4, Nos. 2230–2 (the first of these works is evidently a Central Asian copy from the late eighteenth or early nineteenth century, but Nos. 2231 and 2232 are seventeenth-century copies produced in Iran but brought to Central Asia; the former, 2231, is a work on the anatomy of the brain and the head), 217–20, Nos. 2269–73 (including one manuscript, containing the seventeenth-century *Tuḥfat al-mu'minīn*, copied in 1225/1810 in 'Yanghī Qūrghān' by Mullā Mīr Ni'mat-jān b. Dāmullā Mullā Mīr 'Abd-i Muḥammad [*sic*] Tāshkandī, in 518 ff., No. 2272). On a later Iranian work circulated widely in Central Asia, see Häsäniy (1993, 207–23).
35. See the description of the Central Asian copy of a Persian medical work written for Aḥmad Shāh Durrānī (*KVR*, VI, 198–9, No. 2239), and the description of a likely Central Asian copy, from 1290/1873–4, of a Persian medical work written in 1199/1785 for his son Tīmūr Shāh (*SVR*, IX, 331–3, No. 6501). A later Persian work produced, evidently, in Kabul (in 1220/1805–6), the *Navādir al-favā'id va majma' al-javāhir* of Muṣṭafā b. Muḥammad Ibrāhīm al-Khurāsānī, dedicated to his teacher Sa'd al-Dīn Aḥmad Anṣārī (from a village near Kābul), is represented by four copies in Tashkent (*SVR*, I, 276–7, Nos. 617–20), of which one was clearly copied in Bukhārā (in 1292/1875, No. 618, in 235 ff.), and another is of probable Central Asian origin (No. 620, in 342 ff., copied in 1279/1862–3 by Niyāz-Muḥammad Qarshīgī); the work is of potential interest for the religious dimensions of healing, insofar as it includes, according to the catalogue description, discussions of 'sympathetic and magical means' for curing illnesses in addition to medicines.
36. The Tashkent collection holds two copies of an anonymous Arabic rendering of the work of Paracelsus (d. 1541), one copied in Kazan around 1809 (Inv. No. 3508, *SVR*, I, 277–8, No. 621), the other copied in 1299/1881–2 in Bukhārā and owned by the same Sayyid Mīr Ṣiddīq b. Sayyid Amīr Muẓaffar, whose seal in this case is dated 1296/1878–9 (Inv. No. 2631/III, *SVR*, I, 278, No. 622). Persian translations of French medical works on pediatrics and on the circulation of the blood are preserved in Dushanbe (*KVR*, VI, 202–3, Nos. 2244–5), though they were evidently copied in Iran (in 1296/1879).
37. The work of 'Ḥasrat' is preserved in MS Tashkent, 2905/II (ff. 155b–324a, copied 1261/1844–5 by Ḥājjī Muḥammad Samarqandī), *SVR*, I, 274–5, No. 614; the catalogue description assigns the work the title *Niẓām-i ṣiḥḥat*, and describes it as poetic description of the symptoms of various illnesses written in 1188/1774 by an anonymous native of Marv. The work was noted, as anonymous, in Storey (1971, 278). The same title and manuscript are mentioned in Hikmätulläev (1994, 96), where the author is identified as Sayyid Muḥammad 'Ḥasrat', who served at the court of Bayrām-'Alī Khān in Marv and was killed in 1786. The fullest discussion of 'Ḥasrat' is that of Häsäniy (1993, 112–15), who stresses the paucity of biographical information on the author (without referring to the death-date given by Hikmätulläev), and gives a more detailed account of the work's structure: according to Häsäniy, the manuscript contains two sections of a work originally intended to consist of three parts (the third does not survive or was perhaps never completed); the first section bears the title *Niẓām-i ṣiḥḥat* and was dedicated to Bayrām-'Alī Khān, while the second was dedicated to this ruler's son, Ḥusayn, and bears the separate title *Tuḥfa-yi Ḥusaynī*. Extensive excerpts from the unique manuscript are given in Uzbek translation in Häsäniy (1993, 115–32 [from the first part, and 132–74 [from the second]).
38. MSS Tashkent, 2850/II, ff. 49b–309a, copied 1306/1888 (*SVR*, I, 288, No. 652), called *'Amal al-ṣāliḥīn*; 3490, 427 ff., copied 1250/1834–5 (*SVR*, IX, 374–5, No. 6549; here the cataloguer, Hikmätulläev, inexplicably links the *nisba* Qā'inī with a town of Kurdistan rather than with the well-known town of Khurāsān); 3486, 574 ff., copied in the Dār al-shifā *madrasa* in Bukhārā in 1267/1851 (*SVR*, IX, 375–6, No. 6550); 3493, 468 ff., copied 1268/1851–2 (*SVR*, IX, 376, No. 6551). This work was evidently lithographed in Tehran in 1867; on the author, Ṣāliḥ Qandahārī Qā'inī, see Storey (1971, 279).
39. MS Tashkent, 431, 501 ff., copied 1260/1844 (*SVR*, I, 288–9, No. 653), bearing the seal of Sayyid Mīr Ṣiddīq b. Amīr Muẓaffar; another copy, Inv. No. 2116/VII, is written in the margins of a copy of the fifteenth-century *Anvār-i suhaylī*, at ff. 830b–1004a (*SVR*, I, 289, No. 654).
40. MS Tashkent, 2785, in 158 ff., ascribed to the mid-nineteenth century (*SVR*, I, 275, No. 615).
41. MS Tashkent, 2612/I, ff. 1b–56a, copied in 1275/1858 from a manuscript copied from the author's autograph (*SVR*, I, 275–6, No. 616); this work alone is noted, on the basis of this copy, in Hikmätulläev

(1994, 96–7). Another manuscript of the work is preserved in Dushanbe, Inv. No. 75/II, ff. 59b–124a, copied 1257/1841 (*KVR*, VI, 200, No. 2241).

42. MS Tashkent, 2529/I (1b–16a, ascribed to the late nineteenth century), *SVR*, I, 280, No. 632.
43. MS Tashkent, 2900/XXXII, ff. 483b–498a, copied 1215/1800), *SVR*, V, 291, No. 3959.
44. MS Tashkent, 2716/II (ff. 113b–336a), *SVR*, V, 281, No. 3940.
45. A large copy of the *Ṭibb-i Akbar*, completed in 1112/1700–1 by the Indian author Muḥammad Akbar, known as Arzānī, as a Persian translation and expansion of the work presented by Nafīs b. 'Avaż Kirmānī to Ulugh Beg (see above, note 6), was prepared for Naṣrullāh: MS Tashkent, 4759 (534 ff., copied 1275/1858–9; *SVR*, IX, 324–5, No. 6490). Of uncertain patronage is a copy of the *Shifā' al-maraż*, a medical work in Persian verse by Shihāb al-Dīn b. 'Abd al-Karīm (a native of Ghazna who was evidently trained in medicine in Kabul and wrote his work most likely in 990/1582, in India), completed in Kesh (Shahrisabz), in the *khānqāh* of Shaykh Shams al-Dīn (that is, Kulāl), evidently in 1276/1860 (MS Tashkent, 10,425/II, ff. 9b–122b, described in *SVR*, IX, 311, No. 6478, where the date of copying is given as 25 Shavvāl 1267/16 May 1860, a clear error: 25 Shavvāl 1276 does correspond to 16 May 1860); two other copies are described in *SVR*, IX, 310–11, Nos. 6476–7. Substantial excerpts from the *Shifā' al-maraż* are given in Uzbek translation in Häsäniy (1993, 14–46; Häsäniy says that the Tashkent collection contains two copies of the work, and ascribes the author to the fourteenth century, based on the manuscript described at No. 6476).
46. MS Tashkent, 2906, 483 ff., evidently the author's own copy, or perhaps his draft (*SVR*, I, 267–8, No. 601); cf. Hikmätulläev (1994, 103). For copies of the *Mīzān al-ṭibb* itself, see *SVR*, I, 266–7, Nos. 599–600, and *KVR*, VI, 194–5, No. 2233, with further references to catalogues of collections outside Central Asia.
47. MS Tashkent, 2716/IV, ff. 344b–363a, dated 1255/1839 (*SVR*, I, 290–1, No. 659; the other 'copy', described at *SVR*, I, 291, No. 660, runs to just six folios); noted in Storey (1971, 293).
48. MS Tashkent, 436/VII, ff. 130b–154b, *SVR*, I, 279, No. 627.
49. MS Tashkent, 9254, several parts noted in *SVR*, VIII, 111–13, Nos. 5690–3.
50. On his copy of Subḥān Qulī Khān's work, see above, note 30. Mīr Ṣiddīq's seals appear also in MS Tashkent, 2128/II (ff. 3a–112b), an undated but evidently seventeenth-century copy of the Persian *Zubda-yi qavānīn-i 'ilāj*, written in 871/1466 by Muḥammad b. 'Alā' al-Dīn b. Haybatullāh al-Sabzavārī, known as '*ghiyāth al-mutaṭabbib*' (*SVR*, I, 257, No. 569); on the work and its author, see Storey (1971, 228). Hikmätulläev (1994, 76) refers to a sixteenth-century copy of the same work, in 104 ff., held in the Tashkent collection, evidently not described in the published catalogue, and mentions the seventeenth-century copy in 110 ff., without noting its connection to Mīr Ṣiddīq.
51. MS Tashkent, 254/I (ff. 5b–16b), *SVR*, I, 287, No. 650; the work from which the excerpt is taken is the *Qarābādīn-i Qādirī* of Muḥammad Akbar (Arzānī), written in 1126/1714.
52. MSS Tashkent, 2745/I (1b–83b, 1304/1887; *SVR*, V, 284, No. 3949); 5021/II (5b–145a, 1311/1893; *SVR*, IX, 341–2, No. 6514). Cf. Hikmätulläev (1994, 102–3). Note also the many brief nineteenth-century compilations of 'recipes' for medicines and other therapies, described in *SVR*, I, 279, Nos. 624–6, and V, 281–3, Nos. 3941–6, 284–5, Nos. 3950–3, 291–2, Nos. 3960–3.
53. MS Tashkent, 2572/XXXIV, ff. 770a–787b [*sic*], but also described as comprising eight folios, and hence perhaps 770a–777b), *SVR*, V, 283, No. 3947.
54. MS Tashkent, 2974/II (ff. 108b–219b), *SVR*, I, 278, No. 623; noted in Storey (1971, 291).
55. MS Tashkent, 8257/IX, ff. 45b–54a; *SVR*, VII, 305, No 5468.
56. MS Tashkent, 10,814 (155 ff., copied 1321/1903–4), *SVR*, IX, 345–8, No. 6519; see the extensive description of the work's contents.
57. MS Dushanbe, Inv. No. 1175 (86 ff., evidently copied in 1330/1912), *KVR*, VI, 203–4, No. 2246.
58. Ḥādhiq's *Taḥqīq al-qavā'id* is preserved in three copies in Tashkent, described in *SVR*, IX, 335–8, Nos. 6505–7 (with a detailed description of its contents at No. 6506): Inv. Nos. 6794 (193 ff., copied 1282/1865–6); 1306 (232 ff., copied 1317/1899); and 710 (incomplete, in 90 ff., undated but bearing a seal of Yūnus-jān Dāda Muḥammad-oghlī aghālïq Khūqandī, dated 1338/1919–20). The descriptions are by Hikmätulläev, who wrote a brief article on this author's medical works: Hikmätulläev (1969); see also the discussion in Hikmätulläev (1994, 99–102). Ḥādhiq was a son of the controversial Sufi shaykh known as Islām Shaykh or Ṣūfī Islām (expelled from Bukhārā under Shāh Murād and later killed during the Qājār attack on Herat in 1807). On other Persian translations of Chaghmīnī's *Qānūncha*, see Storey (1971, 219–20).
59. See *SVR*, VII, 300–1, Nos. 5457–9 (5457 = Inv. No. 10,196/III, ff. 95a–209a, copied in 1263/1846–7).

60. MS Tashkent, 12,535/III; this manuscript (not mentioned in *SVR*, but noted in Hikmätulläev [1994, 104–5]), was copied, according to Hikmätulläev, by Ḥāmid-khān Shāshī, the older brother of Bāsiṭ-khān, in 1953 (on these two figures, see below, notes 64–6).
61. One manuscript of this work (in which the author is identified as Maḥmūd Ḥakīm Yayfānī b. Dāmullā Shādī Muḥammad Farghānī), copied in 1356/1937, is preserved in Dushanbe (Inv. No. 1220, in 38 ff.; *KVR*, I, 133–4, No. 132, giving the author's *nisba* as 'Sayfānī'), while another, running to 55 ff. and preserved in a provincial library in Bukhara, was mentioned in McChesney (1978, 24).
62. The lithographed translation is mentioned in the catalogue description of the Khwārazmian translation noted earlier (*SVR*, VII, 292, No. 5448); cf. Hikmätulläev (1994, 116–17), and Häsäniy (1993, 49–50). For a modern Uzbek translation of the *Jāmi' al-favā'id*, or *Ṭibb-i Yūsufī*, based on 'several manuscripts' and printed versions, see Häsäniy (1992); excerpts appear in Häsäniy (1993, 193–204).
63. MS Tashkent, 11083 (125 ff., copied by Shukūr qārī Ātā Khwāja Īshān oghli in 1344/1925–6), *SVR*, VII, 284–7, No. 5444. On the author (who died ca. 1930) and this work, see Hikmätulläev (1994, 114–16).
64. See Hikmätulläev (1994, 106–7); the younger brother also completed an 'Uzbek' translation of Ḥunayn b. Isḥāq's Arabic translation of the aphorisms of Buqrāṭ (that is, Hippocrates; on Persian renderings of the Arabic version, see Storey [1971, 193–4]), but Hikmätulläev makes no mention of a manuscript copy.
65. This work was published, in Cyrillic Uzbek transcription, as Häsäniy (2003).
66. These works are mentioned in Hikmätulläev (1994, 107–9), with no further particulars on the whereabouts of the manuscripts; presumably they are in the Tashkent collection, or still in private hands.
67. A fuller picture of the extent of Islamic medical literature produced in Central Asia will be possible when the current project to prepare an online catalogue of the Beruni institute's manuscripts is completed.

References

Allworth, Edward A., and Rustam Shukurov. 2004. *The Personal History of a Bukharan Intellectual: The Diary of Muḥammad-Sharīf-i Ṣadr-i Ziyā*. Leiden: Brill.

Beckwith, Christopher I. 2009. *Empires of the Silk Road: A History of Central Eurasia from the Bronze Age to the Present*. Princeton: Princeton University Press.

DeWeese, Devin. 2011. "Survival Strategies: Reflections on the Notion of Religious 'Survivals' in Soviet Ethnographic Studies of Muslim Religious Life in Central Asia." In *Exploring the Edge of Empire: Soviet Era Anthropology in the Caucasus and Central Asia*, edited by Florian Mühlfried and Sergey Sokolovskiy, 35–58. Münster: Lit Verlag.

Fonahn, Adolf. 1910. *Zur Quellenkunde der persischen Medizin*. Leipzig: J. A. Barth.

Gallagher, Nancy. 2012. "Medicine and Modernity in the Middle East and North Africa." *International Journal of Middle East Studies* 44: 799–807.

Ḥāfiẓ Tanïsh. 1983. *Khafiz-i Tanysh ibn Mir Mukhammad Bukhari, Sharaf-nama-ii shakhi (Kniga shakhskoi slavy)*. Translated by M. A. Salakhetdinova. Moscow: Nauka, ch. 1.

Häsäniy, Mähmud, trans. 1991. *Häkim Dävaiy äl-Gilaniy: Fävayidu-l-insan ('insanlärgä faydälär')*. Tashkent: Mäjnuntal.

Häsäniy, Mähmud, trans. 1992. *Baburning khas täbibi Yusufiy täbabäti*. Tashkent: Fän.

Häsäniy, Mähmud. 1993. *Täbabät durdanäläri*. Tashkent: Ibn Sina namidägi näshriyat-mätbäa birläshmäsi.

Häsäniy, Mähmud, ed. 2003. Basitkhan ibn Zahidkhan Shashii, *Qanuni Basitiy*. 2 vols. Tashkent: Fän.

Häsäniy, Mähmud, and Nuri Yoldasheva, eds. 1994. *as-Sä'idu-s-Sämärqändiy: Janzatlärning tibbiy khasiyätläri*. Tashkent: Fän.

Hikmätulläev, H. 1969. "Shair Haziqning tibbiy äsärläri vä täbibligi häqidä." *Ozbek tili vä ädäbiyati* 3: 50–52.

Hikmätulläev, Hämidullä. 1994. *Shärq täbabäti*. Tashkent: Äbdullä Qadiriy namidägi Khälq Merasi Näshriyati.

Hofman, H. F. 1969. *Turkish Literature: A Bio-Bibliographical Survey*, Section III (Chaghatai), Part I (Authors). Utrecht: University of Utrecht.

KVR: *Katalog vostochnykh rukopisei Akademii nauk Tadzhikskoi SSR*, edited by A. M. Mirzoev and A. E. Bertels, vol. VI. Dushanbe: Donish, 1988.

László, Károly. 2006. "A Seventeenth-Century Chaghatay Treatise on Medicine." In *Orvostörténeti Közlemények/Communicationes de historia artis medicinae* (Budapest), 194–195: 51–61.

Levey, Martin, and Noury al-Khaledy, trans. 1967. *The Medical Formulary of Al-Samarqandi and the Relation of Early Arabic Simples to Those Found in the Indigenous Medicine of the Near East and India*. Philadelphia: University of Pennsylvania Press.

McChesney, R. D. 1978. "A Guide to Orientalist Research in Soviet Central Asia." *MESA Bulletin* 12 (1): 13–25.

Michaels, Paula A. 2003. *Curative Powers: Medicine and Empire in Stalin's Central Asia*. Pittsburgh: University of Pittsburgh Press.

Miklukho-Maklai, N. D., ed. 1964. *Persidskie i tadzhikskie rukopisi Instituta narodov Azii AN SSSR (Kratkii alfavitnyi katalog)*. Moscow: Nauka, ch. 1.

Rieu, Charles. 1881. *Catalogue of the Persian Manuscripts in the British Museum,* Vol. II. London: British Museum.

Savage-Smith, Emilie. 2000. "Ṭibb." *Encyclopaedia of Islam,* New Edition X: 452–460. Leiden: Brill.

Sezgin, Fuat. 1970. *Geschichte des arabischen Schrifttums: Medizin – Pharmazie – Zoologie – Tierheilkunde*. Leiden: Brill.

Shterenshis, M. V. 2000. "Oriental Medical Manuscripts in Uzbekistan: An Overview." *Vesalius* 6 (2): 100–104.

Storey, C. A. 1971. *Persian Literature: A Bio-Bibliographical Survey,* Vol. II, Part 2, E. *Medicine*. London: Luzac & Co.

SVR: *Sobranie vostochnykh rukopisei Akademii nauk Uzbekskoi SSR*, edited by A. A. Semenov *et al.* Tashkent: Fan, 1952–87.

Vámbéry, Herrmann. 1867. *Ćagataische Sprachstudien*. Leipzig: F. A. Brockhaus.

Vokhidov, Shodmon, and Zoir Choriev. 2007. *Sadr-i Ziia i ego biblioteka (Iz istorii knigi i knizhnoi kul'tury v Bukhare v nachale XX veka)*, kniga 1. Tashkent: Yängi äsr ävladi.

The opium war at the 'roof of the world': the 'elimination' of addiction in Soviet Badakhshan

Alisher Latypov[a,b]

[a]*The Central Asia Program, Institute for European, Russian, and Eurasian Studies, The Elliott School of International Affairs, George Washington University, Washington, DC, USA;* [b]*Global Health Research Center of Central Asia (GHRCCA), Columbia University, New York, NY, USA*

This article provides an overview of drug consumption in the Pamirs in the late nineteenth and early twentieth centuries and examines the evolution of the early Soviet responses to opium smoking in Soviet Badakhshan on the basis of published literature, archival materials, oral histories and medical records. The author demonstrates that biomedicine remained significantly underdeveloped in that region during the first decades of Soviet rule, with central and local authorities relying on punitive and restrictive administrative measures in their fight against drug addiction. As these measures failed to wipe out opiate addiction in Gorno-Badakhshan, the opium war at the 'roof of the world' culminated in the Great Terror, providing the Stalinist regime with the 'radical' solution by liquidating drug dealers without any 'show trials' and incarcerating opiate consumers. The consequences of such administrative regulation of addiction in Soviet Badakhshan were dire: in the years between 1941 and 1968, only few patients with the diagnosis of *narkomania* were hospitalized in the Tajik Republican Psychiatric Hospital, while the exact numbers of repressed drug users who perished in prisons and Gulag camps are destined to remain unknown.

Introduction

In many parts of pre-Soviet Central Asia, teahouses were the most popular places for male entertainment and socialization over a tasty meal and a bowl of tea. Offering some rest in the shadow of trees during spring and summer and the warmth of fire on a cold winter day, teahouses also served as common sites for both the consumption and sale of opiates and other products containing narcotic substances. The 'liquidation' of these private outlets by the Bolsheviks and the opening of new, red teahouses (*krasnye chaikhany*) have been linked by Soviet authors with conquering drug addiction in this region (Antsyferov 1934; Guliamov 1980, 1988; Guliamov and Pogosov 1987; Gulomov, Sharofov, and Kleandrov 1989).

In Soviet Tajikistan, no psychiatric hospital was operational until 1941, whereas the first specialized narcological facility (*kabinet*) was opened only in the late 1950s. Although the first 10 psychiatric beds were established in the infectious-diseases hospital sometime around the mid-1930s in the capital city of Tajikistan, they did not serve drug-treatment purposes and were designated for the temporary sedation and restraint of patients with acute psychiatric conditions (Latypov 2010, 2011b). In view of the above situation, there was a common belief among Soviet Tajik psychiatrists and narcologists that until the 1940s, Tajik drug addicts were sent for specialized treatment to other psychiatric facilities located outside of the country, particularly to Uzbekistan. This assertion was replicated in numerous publications and was particularly encouraged since it served to sustain the image of the benevolent Soviet state and its biomedicine project, which took care of the sick addicts and was even willing to refer them for treatment to other republics (Guliamov 1987; Guliamov and Subbotin 1972, 1984).

The actual situation with regard to drug-prevention and addiction treatment in Tajikistan in the 1920s and 1930s was far more complex and differed dramatically from its official description by Soviet authors. As I have shown in my recent research, in the 1920s and 1930s, only a very small number of patients with opiate addiction received specialized drug-dependence treatment at local and regional biomedical establishments, and the prevention of drug use among Tajiks by means of a network of red teahouses was as true as many other myths invented during the Soviet era (Latypov 2011a, 2011b). These statements, however, raise a question of vital importance for our understanding of the administration of addiction in Soviet Tajikistan. If the majority of local opiate users were left untreated and if red teahouses did not prevent the consumption of narcotics by the local population, how, in fact, did the Soviet regime 'eliminate' drug use in early Soviet Tajikistan? In this paper, I will aim to answer this question by first looking at the historical context of opium use in the Pamirs as well as the early biomedical interventions of the Soviet regime in that region, and then providing a detailed account of the administrative 'opium war' that took place in Soviet Badakhshan and ended with repressions during Stalin's Great Terror in 1936–9.[1]

Opium use in the Pamirs in the late nineteenth and early twentieth centuries

Long before Soviet rule was established in the Pamirs, a Danish military officer and explorer visiting the region at the turn of the nineteenth and twentieth centuries observed heavy use of opium by the natives. Ole Olufsen travelled to the Pamirs on several occasions and in his 1900 publication wrote that 'in his time practically every household cultivated poppy (*kuknar*) in their own garden and that many people used opium (*afiun*) themselves: it was either smoked or else the capsules were ground to powder and dissolved in water' (Bliss 2006, 164–165). Four years later he was more specific and stated that these were only the poor who smoked opium in Vakhan, in sharp contrast to Shugnan and Garan, where 'all classes' were given to the smoking of opium. As for opium poppy, it was the plant 'never wanting in the gardens of natives' (Olufsen 1904, 120–121). After Russia gained a formal right to deploy its frontier posts in the Western Pamirs as part of the Anglo-Russian frontier agreement in 1895, the reports of the Russian military doctors began to portray a more detailed picture of the use of opium by the local population. In 1903, a senior doctor of the Pamir detachment in Khorog, Propaschikh (1903) published his article in *Turkestanskie Vedomosti* focusing on opium use in Vakhan, Shugnan and Rushan areas. Echoing Olufsen, he confirmed that in remote Vakhan only few people used opium whereas inhabitants of Rushan and Shugnan seemed to be significantly affected by this 'pernicious habit', with opium use being particularly widespread in Khorog and Porshnev villages. Although opium was mostly supplied from the neighbouring Afghan province of Ishkashim and the city of Faizabad, nearly every household in the region allocated some plot for opium-poppy cultivation, which was not necessarily and not primarily for domestic consumption, but rather for some sort of 'exploitation' of other opium users that the author did not specify. Briefly mentioning the period between the twelfth and late nineteenth centuries when, 'as the legend says', Tajiks got their first exposure to opium through the local elites, Propaschikh identified two main 'culprits' to blame for the chilling situation that he witnessed: the Afghan and Bukharan rulers. Being in charge of the region from the early 1880s until mid-1890s and themselves prone to opium use 'due to the proximity to the British India', Afghans supposedly did not prohibit narcotics consumption in their temporarily acquired territories and by doing so they 'further spread the use of opium among the local Tajiks' (263). As for Bukharan authorities, who formally administered those territories following the Anglo-Russian border settlement of 1895, they did not pay any attention to drug use among the natives either and often shared this habit with Pamiri people. In the latter case, as Propaschikh believed, it was ostensibly the proximity to the main Bukharan dominions that made Rushan and Shugnan areas vulnerable in terms of opium use to such an extent that 'in the last 7–8 years the use of opium became so deeply rooted among the Tajiks, especially the residents of the two abovementioned villages, that women too started to abuse opium, – something that, according to the natives, had not happened before' (264). According to Propaschikh, smoking was the primary mode of opium consumption in the Pamirs and people usually initiated it at the age of 15 or 16. There was hardly anything he could do to cure those 'desperate subjects', since 'the beginner smokers usually do not seek for Russian health care here, it is the elderly ones, who had smoked for a long time and destroyed their health beyond restoration by any medical intervention, that are after it' (264).

Propaschikh's successor, Dr S. N. Averkiev, who summarized his 17-month practice in Khorog between August 1903 and January 1905 in a lengthy *'etude'* on the medical aid to the Pamiri population, similarly reported that there were only two opium smokers out of a total 411 patients seen by him during that period (Averkiev 1905a, 1905b, 1905c). He attempted to treat one of them with 'persuasion' but it was a failed endeavour as 'after one month break in smoking the patient abandoned himself to his passion almost more than before' (Averkiev 1905c, 985).[2]

In the Pamirs, opium was as expensive as silver in the early twentieth century, with one silver coin buying as much opium as its own weight. On the market, it was valued equally as other vital products, such as rice and tea (Odilbekova 1984; Propaschikh 1903). In 1915–16, a scholar of Pamiri languages, I. I. Zarubin recorded an oral history from one resident of Shugnan called Nagzibek who provided a detailed description of his childhood experiences as a son of an opium smoker. His father had to sell all their property in order to support his habit and in summer times had to work for the Russian frontier detachment as a labourer (*chernorabochii*) for one and a half *tenge* per day. He would spend all his income on opium, letting his family go a-begging (Odilbekova 1984).

After the Turkestan General Governorate in Tashkent declared 'temporary Russian administration' and annexed Vakhan, Shugnan and Rushan in January 1905, the head of the Pamir detachment, Mukhanov, got a free hand to introduce drug prohibition. In 1906, cultivation of opium poppy was prohibited in the Western Pamirs, while the importation of opium from the neighbouring countries as well as 'dissemination' of the opium-smoking habit were made punishable by a fine or arrest. Opium smokers, such as Nagzibek's father, were no longer hired to labour at the Pamir detachment (Iskandarov and Iusupov 1976). In the same year Baron Cherkasov, the secretary of the Russian political agency in Bukhara who was sent to the Pamirs on a socio-economic and political fact-finding mission, wrote in his secret report that 'with time, it would be useful to introduce the placement of [opium] smokers under the guardianship of a rural society, together with the withdrawal of the voting right at the elections and the right to occupy positions in rural administration' (Iskandarov and Iusupov 1976, 39).[3]

However, when in October 1914 colonel Ivan Iagello was made the head of the Pamir detachment, he could see no results of the anti-opium efforts made by his predecessors. In April 1916, Iagello acknowledged that 'opium smoking is sustained and continues to spread with persistent power, bringing to ruin and devastating not only individual persons, but families and entire *kishlak*s as well,' thereby forcing him to issue a decree which granted opium users 20 days for giving up their habit.[4] After this period local *aksakal*s ('white-beards'; elderly informal village leaders) and heads of *volost*s (districts) were required to take 'the most energetic measures', including confiscation of both pipes and opium as well as imposing a 15-rouble fine for every revealed episode of opium smoking. This fine was supposed to be subject to the financial wellbeing of smokers and their ability to pay it. Iagello stayed in his position until 1917 and joined the Bolsheviks when they came to power.

While elsewhere in the Bukhara Emirate and in many other parts of Central Asia opiates were mainly ingested orally as a poppy tea or as all sorts of pills and electuaries, with varying content of opium and for medicinal or recreational reasons, it was the *smoking* of opium as a predominant mode of consumption that made the natives of the Western Pamirs more affected by their drug habit (at this stage, one can only tentatively suggest that the custom of smoking might have spread to the Pamirs from Chinese Turkestan).[5] Despite all the sanctions introduced by the pre-revolutionary Russian military authorities since 1906, it appears that by the time the Soviet rule was consolidated in Gorno-Badakhshan Autonomous Oblast and the newly formed Tajik government could function, the situation with opium use in the Pamirs remained as dramatic, if not worse, as before. As a 'baseline' of the tsarist past that the Communists had to tackle in the Pamirs, Tajik historians suggest the following data: 'Opium smoking was very much spread in the region. It is considered that up to 60% of the population was overwhelmed by this disease. Some households spent almost 90% of their income on opium. In some districts and villages the entire population was infected by the illness. Thus, for instance, there was not a single family in Shugnan district where at least one of its members would not smoke opium. In Rushan, opium smoking was nearly universal, with up to 90% of [people's] income being spent on purchasing opium' (Shergaziev 1959, 79).[6] Although any estimate of that kind, made at a time when the Tajik administration could not gather reliable data on even the most basic issues should be interpreted extremely cautiously, it is clear that the smoking of opium in Gorno-Badakhshan could not have passed unnoticed by the Communist regime.

To date, against the backdrop of several published texts that very briefly mention the issue of drugs in Tajikistan in the 1920s, there seems to be only one 'comprehensive' Soviet account of the Bolsheviks' response to opium smoking in the Pamirs. Offered by Pavel Luknitsky, a writer who visited the Pamirs on several occasions and accompanied the 1932 USSR Academy of Sciences' Comprehensive Expedition to Tajikistan as a Scientific Secretary, this account offers a straightforward description, or rather another myth that until now remained unchallenged, of a scene that greeted the Bolsheviks when they arrived on Pamiri soil and how that scene was then transformed forever:

> Everything had to be created from the very beginning. Not a single cart could travel over the toothed, knife-edge tracks in Western Pamir. The Kirghiz of Murgab treated toothache with red-hot nails and rubbed a mixture of ashes, dung and mutton fat into open wounds. The women did not know the use of scissors, and many of the highlanders had never seen window glass. People with huge goiters wandered about in Vanch and Yazgulem. The people's minds were filled with horrible superstitions.
>
> Opium smoking drove people to insanity …
> The year 1925 was an eventful one for Badakhshan. At the end of the year the First Pamir Congress of Soviets was held in Khorog, and [in its aftermath] people became aware, from the effect it had upon themselves, that the Soviet Government had launched a vigorous campaign against hunger, the miserable standard of living, opium smoking and disease … Party organizers went to the most remote *kishlaks* and rallied the poor peasantry for the fight against their class enemies, organized assistance of every kind for the population, and disbursed long-term loans to the needy.
>
> In 1931 the first regular detachment of the Soviet Frontier Guards arrived in Western Pamir, and since then the green trimming of their uniforms has been dear to the hearts of all the inhabitants of Badakhshan … Smuggling was stopped, so also was opium smoking. Scores of doctors and midwives performed their beneficial functions in newly built hospitals and dispensaries in Ishkashim, Murgab, Kalai-Vamar, Bartang and Vanch. They restored sight to the blind who came from

> Afghanistan. Smallpox vanished; malaria declined; there were no new cases of leprosy ... This is how, vanquishing the wild mountains and age-long ignorance, surmounting thousands of barriers of different kinds, Soviet rule was strengthened and transformed the life in Pamir during those ten years! (Luknitsky 1954, 233–237)

However, as one looks back at this account through the prism of contemporary records, many facets of it turn out to have their own, far more complex stories. When combined, they cast a different light on the above transformations in early Soviet Badakhshan and uncover multiple areas of the Communists' struggle against drug addiction, the failure of the Soviet doctor in this struggle, and an ultimate 'elimination' of *narkomania* in Tajikistan by the organs of power in the 1930s.

Biomedical response to *narkomania* in Soviet Badakhshan

That Luknitsky juxtaposed opium smoking against 'beneficial functions' of doctors in the Pamirs was not a coincidence. Despite the strategic location of the Gorno-Badakhshan Autonomous Oblast often considered as a 'red light' at the crossroads of Afghanistan, China and India, biomedicine remained significantly underdeveloped in this remote area throughout the period between the 1920s and 1950s. While health-care assistance to opium users was barely available locally, there was also no road connection with the capital of Tajikistan until 1940 to allow speedy access to medical assistance beyond the region. Travelling on horse was possible only in some sections along the route and only for a limited period of time during the year, often taking weeks and even months before one would reach the centre.

In November 1925, when the First Pamir Congress of Soviets determined to launch an immediate and most energetic struggle against opium smoking and obliged the *oblast*'s medical personnel to conduct broad sanitary-enlightenment activities both among the general population and opium smokers, human resources in public health were almost non-existent in Gorno-Badakhshan. Until 1924, when the first outpatient unit staffed with civilian health workers was established in GBAO, all biomedical assistance to the local residents was provided by the military medical personnel of the frontier detachments. Following the 1925 Congress, the first 15-bed hospital was founded in Khorog along with three outpatient units in Rushan, Murgab and Ishkashim. By the mid-1928, the entire region (inhabited by some 28,374 people as of 1926) covering nearly half of the Tajik ASSR's territory had only two hospitals with an overall capacity of 25 beds as well as three medical points.[7] According to some records, these institutions were staffed by three doctors including one dentist as well as seven *fel'dsher*s (health-care professionals working mainly in the field) (Aknazarov 2005b; Mirzobekov 1974; Nazarshoev 1982).

However, at that time some medical workers seemed to have paid scant attention to opium smoking in the Pamirs and more to indulging in other types of activities. In his report on the state of public health in Autonomous Gorno-Badakhshan Oblast delivered at the People's Commissariat of Public Health's (Narkomzdrav) meeting on 29 March 1932 and published in the first-ever issue of the *Zdravookhranenie Tadzhikistana* (Public Health of Tajikistan) journal, the deputy chief of the public-health administration for Gorno-Badakhshan, Nikolai Tel'iants, claimed that until 1928, 'drunkenness, troublemaking, and playing cards were thriving among doctors' in the region (Tal'iants 1933, 82).[8] Similarly, when reviewing the results of anti-opium-smoking activities undertaken between April and August 1928, the authorities in Badakhshan pointed to the inability of sanitary-enlightenment organizations to 'struggle' against opium smoking.[9] In April 1928, some Communist leaders in Dushanbe also realized that the region had so far 'escaped from the field of vision' of both the Tajik government and the Party, and decided to send a special commission to collect 'exhaustive materials' on the economic and political situation in Gorno-Badakhshan. Apart from the representatives of the Tajik ASSR Central Executive

Committee, the Organizational Unit of the Communist Party, and the People's Commissariat for Enlightenment (who, according to the provisional arrangements, consisted of Nustratullo Maksum, Gotfrid and Dailiami), this commission also included Dr Verbitsky. The delegation was expected to depart for Badakhshan on 10 May; three days earlier the Tajik Narkomzdrav approved the plan of Verbitsky's survey, which consisted of 11 subject areas including the analysis of *narkomania* in the region.[10] Verbitsky's mission report was discussed at the Narkomzdrav's meeting on 26 July 1928. Although it primarily prompted the Dushanbe-based administration to develop the measures against smallpox for the following year, Narkomzdrav was also urged to re-consider its staff selection and allocation practices and replace the medical personnel of GBAO by autumn 1928 with a new team headed by the 'young Soviet doctor' Mil'berg (Tal'iants 1933, 82).[11]

Mil'berg stayed in Khorog for less than two years, and when the next group of 12 medical workers arrived in Gorno-Badakhshan in late 1930, they discovered that the regional health administration was headed by a certain *fel'dsher,* Bezrodnyi (Teliiants 1974). In their struggle against opium addiction the new management was guided by old data produced in 1926 by Dr Slavnin, who examined 2956 residents of Rushan district and found that 338 of them (11.4%) were opium addicts (Paradoksov 1932, 1933).[12] Despite the fact that this prevalence rate was considerably lower than any other estimate ever suggested by local authorities and external commentators, opium smoking has invariably ranked among the highest priority public-health issues on the GBAO *Oblzdrav's* agenda in those years.[13] Yet the number of these priorities was so vast and the capacities to address them so limited that no drug-treatment-related aspiration has ever been fulfilled in Gorno-Badakhshan. As Tel'iants recalled many years after his service as the *Narkomzdrav* plenipotentiary in the Pamirs between 1930 and 1933, in addition to 'struggling against opiomania' he also had to carry out other 'daily routine' tasks including his surgical practice and 'fighting' against tick fever, syphilis, trachoma and leprosy among others. Besides, he had to fulfil a number of other public duties such as being a deputy chair of the regional court, chief of the cultural section of the regional trade union council and the 'RKI' (Worker–Peasant Inspectorate) inspector (Teliiants 1974, 49).

Although the need to study the matter of drug treatment and to set up compulsory-treatment institutions was raised in the region since 1928, the *Narkomzdrav* administrators in Dushanbe envisioned establishing a narcological dispensary in the Pamirs only by the end of 1932. However, the plan was eventually dropped because of the funding shortages and the parallel pressure on the Tajik *Narkomzdrav* to meet dozens of other targets including containing the spread of rampant infectious diseases, improving mother and child health, and ensuring access to basic medical care beyond the capital city.[14] Meanwhile, one vacancy for a 'narcologist' was created at Rushan hospital at some point before the end of 1932. The vacancy was not filled though, since no such specialists existed in Tajikistan and recruiting one from outside of the republic for a posting at the border with Afghanistan proved impossible despite a promised salary of 575 rubles, excluding other bonuses.[15]

In 1932, the Presidium of the Executive Committee of GBAO characterized the state of the availability of medical cadres in the region as catastrophic and dispatched Tel'iants to Stalinabad, and if needed to Tashkent, 'to recruit medical workers for the region' (Mirzobekov 1974, 7). In the same year, he himself claimed that despite the absence of narcological dispensaries and designated narcologists, doctors were allegedly treating some opium users who wanted 'to get rid of their habit' in the hospitals. However, as he himself admitted, it was merely 'a drop in the ocean' (Tal'iants 1933, 84–85).[16] In March 1931, the Communist Party Secretariat in Dushanbe (renamed to Stalinabad in 1929) also discussed the issue of opium smoking in the Pamirs and requested regional educational authorities 'to conduct a number of lectures and talks among the school-aged children on the topic of opium smoking as a social evil'.[17] However, physicians could not join such conversations and offer their assistance to teachers as the first ever school-based sanitary doctor arrived in Khorog only by November 1934.

Starting from the mid-1930s, the number of hospitals and outpatient facilities in the region increased considerably. As of 1940, Gorno-Badakhshan had nine hospitals with a total of 171 beds, 16 outpatient clinics and another 22 medical points. They were staffed with 18 doctors and 111 nurses and represented a substantial improvement compared to the situation in 1935, when six doctors, 21 nurses and one maternity and childhood protection inspector worked in the region (Nazarshoev 1982).[18] This expansion coincided with major raises in payments to the medical staff posted in GBAO, who were entitled to a 30% salary increase following the joint resolution of the Tajik SSR Council of People's Commissars and the Central Committee of the Communist Party of Tajikistan as of 3 April 1936. In 1939, an additional 50% increase, authorized by the Tajik SSR Council of People's Commissars with the aim of attracting and retaining qualified cadres in GBAO, made the salaries of health-care workers in the Pamirs some of the most attractive in the country.[19] However, these initial gains achieved before the Second World War did not lead to the establishment of specialist services for opiate users in the Pamirs. In the 1930s, the state's reliance on repressive measures was seen as an appropriate approach to 'deviant minorities' and other 'enemies of the people', culminating in the Great Terror that swept across the USSR. With the war came a major re-allocation of medical personnel and supplies towards the care of wounded soldiers that was concentrated in the capital of the republic. During the war years, four out of eight district-level hospitals in Gorno-Badakhshan were staffed with one doctor while the remaining four did not have any doctors at all. Only slightly more than half of the available vacancies of supporting medical staff were filled (Davliat'erov 1974).

In the first years after the war the Tajik government made an attempt to ameliorate the staff shortages and sent 35 doctors and 100 nurses to GBAO between 1944 and 1948. However, the influx of cadres was paralleled by a massive outmigration of medical personnel from the Pamirs, with 36 doctors and 44 mid-level health workers leaving the region during the same period (Davliat'erov 1974). By the start of 1954, Gorno-Badakshan did not have a single native Pamiri doctor yet and almost all of them were Slavs.[20] While doctors celebrated the accomplishments of the Soviet rule achieved by the thirtieth anniversary of GBAO, an appalling picture was hidden behind the rising figures that were cited in the public discourse as a proof of miraculous transformations in the life of the Pamiris. Indeed, as Shansky wrote in the 1954 November–December issue of *Zdravookhranenie Tadzhikistana*, the number of doctors in Soviet Badakhshan nearly doubled when compared to 1940, and the number of nurses might have increased 12 fold since 1929 (Shansky 1954). However, on 14 September 1954, he was present at the meeting of the then Ministry of Health of the Tajik SSR, where a completely different interpretation was provided with regard to the state of public health in GBAO. In the preceding 20 months, the arrival of new personnel to the Pamirs was dragging far behind the outmigration, with 19 doctors departing and only six new doctors sent to the region. Overall, of some 90.5 physician vacancies only 57.5 were filled by a total of 32 doctors. Most of them, as becomes clear from these statistics, were doing two full-time jobs (*stavki*) at a time. Of these 32 doctors, 26(!) worked in the regional capital city of Khorog, while Rushan and Rosht-Kala districts had no doctors at all, Murgab and Shugnan had one, and Ishkashim had three. Because human resources were so heavily concentrated in Khorog, beds in the remaining eight district hospitals were barely occupied by some four to eight patients and in one case were found to function as hostel beds. Of six rural pharmacies operating in the region, four were staffed by workers with no pharmaceutical background. Of 37 medical points staffed with midwives and *fel'dshers* only four had their own premises while all the rest were placed in the indigenous ('*tuzemnye*') facilities with earthen floors. Similarly, a number of other medical institutions did not have their own premises, including a medical college for nurses, emergency-aid department, and so on. In the Khorog-based regional hospital, where health care was expected to be better, patients with acute stomach and digestive infection, measles, trachoma, skin and venereal diseases were all lying next to each other in one unit. Even when staffed with personnel and equipped with necessary means, the clinical laboratory of the Khorog hospital did not conduct any biochemical and serological tests, ostensibly because of the lack of due supervision (*trebovatel'nost'*) on the part of the chief doctor.[21]

While these accounts demonstrate that biomedically trained doctors and nurses failed to provide any meaningful health-care support to a considerable population of opiate users in early Soviet Badakhshan, there was still one kind of 'drug-related' service for which they were remembered. Back in the first years of the twentieth century, *fel'dsher* Stepan Kanutovich Khmelevsky arrived in the Pamirs to serve at the Russian frontier detachment under the commandership of the famous Russian officer Andrey Snesarev. He left the Pamirs in 1913 for Aulie-Ata (also known as Dzhambul and Taraz) and came back to Gorno-Badakhshan 13 years later, in 1926. Married to a Pamiri woman, Khmelevsky spoke Tajik and learned many Pamiri languages. The natives reportedly loved Khmelevsky and nicknamed him '*Duhtur Boots*' or the 'little doctor' (Iskandarov and Iusupov 1976, 39–40). Following his return to the Pamirs *Duhtur Boots* resumed his medical career and died many decades later, in January 1950. As Tkhostova wrote about this 'revolutionary *fel'dsher*', none could beat Khmelevsky in delivering legible propaganda messages to the local population, and 'his rhymed verses and couplets on *ishans* and opium addicts were known and sung across all the *kishlaks* of the Pamirs' (Tkhostova 1988, 92–93). Directly put, given that the first drug-treatment facility (*kabinet*) of any kind was established in GBAO as late as in 1982 (Kholdarbekov 1983), it was only Khmelevsky's 'word of mouth' propaganda messages and the like that opiate users received from medical workers in (early) Soviet Badakhshan.

The administrative struggle against *narkomania* and the quest for the 'radical' solution

In the absence of any meaningful biomedical response to opiate use in Gorno-Badakhshan, the state's struggle against this 'social evil' had to rely exclusively on various 'administrative' measures throughout the 1920s and 1930s.[22] These measures were mainly focused on discouraging drug use by adopting a punitive approach and restricting civil and economic rights of drug users. None of these actions, however, helped the regime to 'do away' with drug addiction.

In November 1925, the initial principal decision of the First Pamir Congress of Soviets aiming at countering opium smoking in the region was to seek the prohibition of importation, possession and dealing in opium and to inform the neighbouring Afghan authorities of this policy change. Engaging in the above activities was declared an offence punishable in accordance with Article 97 of the Russian Criminal Code by compulsory labour for a period up to three months. Repeat offenders and those falling under the 'particularly important cases' category could be imprisoned for up to two years. In addition, individuals found guilty of these crimes were subject to exile from the border areas and their property confiscated. While opium use was not criminalized, opium users could be punished in line with Article 89 of the Criminal Code with up to one year of imprisonment for not reporting people who they knew were dealing in opium (Rayner 1925). The Congress participants also agreed that it was necessary to arrange show-court trials of drug dealers in areas severely affected by opium smoking such as Rushan district.[23] By summer 1926, prohibition seemed to be the right answer for the Communist Party members in Gorno-Badakhshan, who called for the continuation of the 'merciless struggle against opium smoking' at their first regional party conference in July 1926 (Nazarshoev 1970, 85–86). At the same time, the Second Plenum of the GBAO Executive

Committee noted with satisfaction the successful implementation of anti-opium smoking measures by the militia in Khorog and demanded that other districts, 'where this social evil exists', strengthen their actions against it as well.[24]

Supported both by the party and the local government, the Pamiri militiamen exceeded all expectations and seized 2026 kilograms of opium in 1927 (which was also a reflection of large-scale opium trade in the region). While these record drug seizures were followed by awards to select officers and the commitment to allocate state funding for developing and sustaining the covert network of informants (*'nelegal'naia' set' osvedomitelei*), they did not seem to reduce opium use (Imomyorbekov 2009).[25] It should be made clear, however, that no reliable baseline figures existed and no follow-up data were gathered in systematic ways during that period. The 'administrative department' of the local executive authority, for example, produced its own estimate of opium use in Gorno-Badakhshan suggesting that as many as 30% of the population were affected in the late 1920s.[26] External political evaluators of the region also felt that they had to say something about the scale of opium use, with these statements being rather general in their nature and pointing to the use of opium across all districts in the region.[27] As medical workers were not in a position to fulfil the task of studying the drug situation in the Pamirs, rural councils (*sel' sovety*) of Shugnan as well as other districts were at some points obliged to compile regular reports with quantitative information on the number of individuals who stopped consuming opium.[28] Unfortunately, it was not possible to locate these reports in the archives. Nonetheless, even if such data were collected, it would most probably represent only some districts and only for a limited period of time. While such data would often be limited to opium smoking alone, it would hardly have any meaning without knowing how this information was collected. We would also be unable to draw conclusions on the actual number of people who did cease opium smoking for longer than a given reporting period. In view of these limitations we can only judge the impact of the administrative struggle with caution and on the basis of the nature of subsequent developments in the opium war and perceptions of the drug situation by some of the actors in this 'struggle'. However, missing from this story are the voices of opium users of the Pamirs, who might have given us if not a more accurate, then a very different perspective.

As soon as the local militia cracked down on the opium trade, it became a highly clandestine activity. With the Tajik–Afghan border wide open and many drug traders coming from Afghanistan, arrests of individual dealers could not significantly disrupt what was a lucrative business for the inhabitants of both the left and right banks of the Piandzh River. 'Under active support and harbouring' provided by the Soviet Badakhshan's opium users for whom opium was a vital commodity, Afghan drug traders became 'uncatchable' for the administrative department.[29] This led to a dramatic decrease in opium seizures in GBAO from over two tons in 1927 to half a ton in 1928, and further down to mere 364 grams in the second quarter of 1930 (Imomyorbekov 2009, 20). Yet smuggling was flourishing in the region judging from the information collected by Dr Korovnikov in the areas of Darvaz and Vandj in 1928, with local Tajik women also playing an active role in the trade and opium being the 'number one' commodity (Korovnikov 1929, 61).

While some districts hoped to intensify and better organize the fight against opium smoking by means of establishing the anti-drug Extraordinary Tripartite Commissions consisting of the head of the district, his deputy and the militia chief, the drug trade did not seem to have diminished. The resolution of Gorno-Badakhshan regional administration adopted at the end of 1928 also revealed that for some drug dealers, the consequences of arrest and show trial were relatively minor, as they were later found to work freely for one of the Soviet trade organizations, Uzbektorg, and almost certainly continued to trade in drugs.[30] In early 1931, the party leaders in Dushanbe urged their GBAO comrades to apply the harshest repressive measures against opium traders and intermediary dealers (*skupschiki*).[31] Despite the local attempts to control the flow of narcotics into the country, the issue of on-going opium trade and consumption in Eastern Tajikistan became of particular concern for the centre in Moscow, when the Political Bureau of the All-Union Communist Party considered the so-called 'Pamirs issue' in June 1931. The Politburo resorted to the political and secret police, the United State Political Directorate (Ob'edinennoe Gosudarstvennoe Politicheskoe Upravlenie, OGPU) as a solution to the 'issue' and requested from this agency to strengthen the struggle against the opium trade.[32] However, the involvement of OGPU and repressive measures against drug dealers did not prove sufficient to curb the supply of drugs. As of the end of March 1932, public-health administrators from GBAO reaffirmed that the struggle against opium addiction continued to be a matter of great urgency and lamented the failure of authorities to come up with a 'radical method' so far (Tal'iants 1933, 84). One year later, in March 1933, the Executive Committee of GBAO had to deal with drug use one more time and issue another resolution on *categorical* [emphasis added] prohibition of use, possession, and trade in opium and cannabis (Imomyorbekov 2009).

In the context of an uninterruptible trade in opium and the lack of drug-treatment institutions in the region, several reports stressed the poor outcomes of the 'struggle against opium smoking' in the late 1920s and early 1930s. They also emphasized the extremely widespread and, on one occasion, increasing use of opium in Gorno-Badakhshan. In an extreme example from Rushan, it was noted that nearly everyone was smoking opium as of September 1930.[33]

The inability of the local militia to cut the supply of opium to the markets and the helplessness of physicians in dealing with drug-dependent residents of the Pamirs resulted in the adoption by both groups of one common goal for the opium war in Soviet Badakhshan: to make the consumption of opium less 'contagious' and visible to the public in order to prevent non-users from initiating opium use. This goal could be achieved by driving opium users underground and forcing them to consume drugs in secrecy. By the end of 1928, the GBAO Executive Committee was already celebrating the initial signs of a shift in the patterns of opium use towards that goal.[34]

Criminalizing drug-related activities and pushing opium smokers away from the streets and communal places should have made the prospects for the near future clear enough for many drug users in the Pamirs. Soviet activists also seemed to have little doubt about the consequences of their anti-drug campaign and proposed to make sure that no drug user crosses the Piandzh River and seeks refuge in Afghanistan, thus undermining the regime's claims to a better life in Soviet Badakhshan.[35] While drug use *per se* was not criminalized, opium smoking represented a major challenge to the regime's agenda of transforming social, economic and political order in the Pamirs. Promising moral and material support to those who would have the strength to give up drugs on their own, Soviet authorities also put every effort to discouraging drug use by 'boycotting' opium smokers in all walks of life. Government organs, public and trade organizations were prohibited from employing opium users. The so-called '*opiists*' (opium users) were denied the right to be elected as members of councils (*sovety*) at any level. When discovered to be elected or employed in the above institutions they were subject to regular purges.[36] Of particular importance to the Communist leaders was to keep opium users clear from the party ranks. Moreover, they also obliged every GBAO Communist Party and Komsomol member to carry out the fight against opium smoking in their families.[37] Between December 1929 and March 1930 the Communist Party of Gorno-Badakhshan underwent the purge that led to the exclusion of 17 members out of a total of 112 people who were checked. Although the majority of the excluded members were blamed for supporting the ideology of the rich men (*baiskaia ideologiia*) and 'merging with the alien element', some were purged for opium smoking and one party member received a strict reprimand (*strogii vygovor*) for 'the poor struggle against opium smoking in one's family'.[38] In the late 1920s, the local authorities of Gorno-Badakhshan also began to set up various public institutions including the anti-opium-smoking society and the *kishlak* commissions for putting opium users under boycott. However, with a significant proportion of the population using drugs, it was rather these commissions who had difficulties in fulfilling their functions and who, instead, found themselves boycotted both by the opium users and the ordinary (non-drug-using) 'citizens'.[39]

Perhaps the most important and troublesome implications of the widespread opium use in the Pamirs for the Bolshevik authorities in the late 1920s were the economic losses of the state and the continuing dependence of the local population on the state credits and loans. According to some statistics, around 30% of all households in the Western Pamirs benefited from state loans in 1925 and 1926, which totalled 30,000 rubles. Information from the Agricultural Bank points to a further 63,776 rubles disbursed between 1927 and 1930. Despite the fact that this financial aid was originally intended to be spent on purchasing live cattle, seeds and agricultural tools as well as the construction of residential houses, the Soviet regime soon discovered that the overwhelming share of all credits had been spent on opium instead.[40] In September 1928 the GBAO Executive Committee confirmed that it would be appropriate to apply 'economic boycotting' against opium users and gave the green light to the district-level committees to implement this policy. On 30 December 1928 the Executive Bureau of the Uzbek Communist Party discussed the results of the Pamirs survey carried out by the Tajik Government's commission and proposed that future credits are provided in kind only, with monetary credits allocated in exceptional circumstances.[41] In September 1930, a politico-economic report on GBAO underlined that agricultural credits were still used to support the opium-smoking habit, although to a lesser extent as compared to the previous years, when local drug users spent up to 90% of whatever resources they had on opium. It was also noted that the non-opium-smokers' households were much better off than the ones belonging to the '*opiists*'.[42] However, some districts, it will be remembered, did not witness any decrease in opium consumption. Moreover, according to one report on '*kolkhoz* construction' process dated 25 September 1930, all members of '*Krasnyi Pamir*' (Red Pamir) kolkhoz in Kurgan-Tube district of Tajikistan were reportedly spending most of their state-allocated credits on opium and cannabis.[43] This almost certainly suggests that at least some 'resettlement' in Kurgan-Tube area was in fact an exile of drug users from the Pamirs – tactics which served the purpose of limiting users' access to drugs as well as making the affected communities 'less infected' with *narkomania*.

As mentioned above, in the early 1930s there was a feeling among GBAO administrators that despite all the measures, they had failed to offer a 'radical' solution to opium smoking. Then, it was the turn of the deputy head of OGPU, Genrikh Iagoda, to raise the 'Pamirs issue' in his special report to Stalin in April 1934.[44] This time it was related to the rise in 'emigrational inclinations' in the Eastern Pamirs orchestrated by the 'counter-revolutionary' group consisting of the former deputy head of the GBAO Executive Committee, who 'crossed the cordon' and left the country in 1933, the former head of Murgab District Executive Committee, the former head of Murgab District Control Commission, the former head of the cultural propaganda unit of the Murgab District Communist Party Committee, and one British resident. According to this report, the dissatisfaction of the population that resulted from the excesses ('*peregib*' or the 'breaches of socialist legality') created favourable conditions for the emergence of counter-revolutionary rumours suggesting that 'the Soviet authorities will conduct mass arrests, seize live cattle, uproot everybody to Russia, and the only escape from this is to flee to Afghanistan.'[45] After studying Iagoda's report, Stalin called for a meeting and put his resolution on the cover page of the report:

> It is necessary to send a battalion of good red army servicemen to the Pamirs and increase the salary of the latter by several times. I. Stalin.[46]

Although I was unable to get access to any further evidence on the subsequent actions by the battalion of 'good' Red Army servicemen in the Pamirs, there is little doubt that there were significant consequences for the residents of GBAO following Stalin's resolution, with opium users and other 'counter-revolutionary elements' targeted in the first place.

In 1936, the Soviet troops tightened control over the border with Afghanistan in anticipation of Stalin's Great Terror. It is likely that because of severe political, administrative and economic pressures some drug users managed to cross the river and escape to Afghani Badakhshan before the frontier was sealed by the iron curtain sometime after late 1937.[47] Others, such as Pamihudo Khushvakhtov from Kalai-Vamar, were able to eventually give up their opium-smoking habit on their own and were later commended by the regime for their hard work (Nazarshoev 1970). Clearly, a certain percentage of the local population was still using drugs when the Great Terror reached the Tajik SSR in late 1937, offering the 'radical' solution to opium smoking in the Pamirs. While open-access materials in Tajik archives are silent on the fate of these people, border regions in Tajikistan were considered 'most affected by the activities of the enemies' and thus were hit especially badly.[48] Oral histories collected from the local residents of Gorno-Badakshan suggest that some drug users were put in prisons in 1937, where they served a term of about 10 years (Keshavjee 1998; personal communication with Maram Azizmamadov, 19 November 2009). For an unknown number of them this was a death sentence.

Although drug users were not specifically mentioned in the NKVD Order No. 00447 'On the Operation on Repressing Former Kulaks, Criminals and Other Anti-Soviet Elements' as of 30 July 1937, there can be little doubt that some of them had a history of having to support their drug habit by stealing or dealing in drugs. They were probably targeted as 'criminals' or – as specified in the NKVD Circular No. 61 issued a week later and providing further explanations in regard to the category 'criminals' for the purposes of repression – they were considered 'criminals without a permanent place of residence, not involved in socially useful labour, against whom no accusation of specific crime is levelled, but who maintain contacts with the criminal community (*kriminal'naia sreda*)' (Iunge, Bordiukov, and Binner 2008, 98–114).[49]

According to the above NKVD Order 00447, the operation on repressing former *kulaks*, criminals and other anti-Soviet elements began in Tajikistan on 10 August 1937. By 2 October 1937, when Andrei Andreev (at that time the secretary of TsK VKP(b)) wrote his report to Stalin from the 'Stalin's city' of Stalinabad, the Chairman of the Tajik People's Council of Commissars Abdullo Rakhimbaev was arrested along with his deputies (according to Nurmukhamedov [1988] , Rakhimbaev was arrested on 9 September 1937). Also arrested were the Chairman of the Tajik Central Executive Committee, his secretary, nearly all People's Commissars and 15 secretaries of the district-level committees. More arrests of 'participants of anti-soviet organization' were under way, including the first and the second secretaries of the Tajik Communist Party, as for Andreev it was obvious that the 'enemies have done a proper job' in Tajikistan and yet were feeling themselves 'quite free'.[50]

As for drug dealers, opium-den owners and smugglers, this time they were repressed without any 'show trials'. Some of the militiamen who, by a cruel irony of fate, were earlier rewarded for their active fight against opium smoking, including Ibragim Ismailov and Ul'fatsho Miralishoev, were arrested and shot as 'enemies of the people' (Imomyorbekov 2009; Motylev 1977). Yet, this was not the end of the opium war at the 'roof of the world', for some of those non-opium-smoking well-off families in Gorno-Badakhshan were also murdered as '*kulaks*' during the Stalinist terror (Bliss 2006). It was perhaps not a coincidence that between 1937 and 1939 Soviet Badakhshan's regional musical and legitimate theatre played 'The Rich and the Opium Smoker', allowing the local viewers to reconsider their future prospects under the Soviet regime (Nazarshoev 1982). What none of them could suspect though, is that Andrei

Andreev, the man who came to Tajikistan in the midst of the Great Terror in order to assess the 'damage' done by the 'enemies' and advise Stalin on 'corrective'/repressive measures, would himself become one of the top-ranking Politburo drug users at some point in his party career, albeit with access to all the medical care he might have needed to treat his drug habit (Zhirnov 2009).[51]

Conclusion

In 1952, after long years of waiting, Pavel Luknitsky's dream of paying one more visit to the Pamirs came true. He travelled around all the districts of the Pamirs except Murgab. In 1955, he wrote that during his last trip he did not see or even hear of anybody smoking opium or hashish on the Soviet side of the Piandzh River (Luknitskii 1955). Indeed, as can be seen from the medical logbooks of the first Tajik Republican [Clinical] Psychiatric Hospital, where patients with the diagnosis of *narkomania* were treated since this asylum became operational in 1941, this time he probably was not mythologizing. Of hundreds of drug-dependent people hospitalized in this institution between 1941 and 1968 there was only one Tajik man and one Russian woman from GBAO.[52] Clearly, the opium war at the 'roof of the world' cost human lives. Yet, it also had profound and far-reaching effects in terms of driving drug users of the Pamirs deep underground and placing many of them in prisons, so that not only visitors like Luknitsky but also medical workers could neither see nor hear about them (Guliamov 1963).

On 19 May 1955, the *Badakhshoni Soveti* (Soviet Badakhshan) newspaper published two articles. The first one, titled 'Medical Care of the Population Ought To Be Improved' and authored by Rakhimov, began with the standard ode to the Communist Party and its constant concern and attention to the issue of public health. However, it also stressed the importance of underlining that 'until now, public health care workers of our [GBAO] region have not organized their activities as required' (Rakhimov 1955, 2). The author of the second article, *kandidat* of medical sciences Ostrovsky, claimed in his opening sentence that 'the life of the workers of our country [Soviet Union] is getting better from year to year', – another standard declaration of the time. 'However', – Ostrovsky noted, 'there are certain habits which are, as surviving vestiges of the past, a great hindrance to this [process]', with the harm of tobacco smoking being the main subject of his article (Ostrovsky 1955, 4). As for the opium war in Soviet Badakhshan, the 'Party organizers', to borrow from Luknitsky, preferred to keep silent on how in fact we have come from the administrative struggle against the scourge of opium smoking in the 1920s to attacking the smoking of cigarettes (*papirosy*) in the 1950s as 'traces of the primitive past'.

Against the backdrop of this silence that continues until the present day, as well as the lack of solid scholarly research on drug histories both in Tajikistan and in other former Soviet republics, this paper aims to fill this gap and to take one of the first steps towards a better understanding of the Communist regime's handling of the 'drug problem' in Soviet Central Asia. As I have argued elsewhere (Latypov 2012), Central Asian drug literature lacks sensitivity to the Soviet historical roots and is abundant in inaccuracies that mislead contemporary drug-control efforts by reinforcing the misrepresentation of drugs in this region as essentially irrelevant until the post-Soviet period. Yet determining when drugs become an issue may be secondary to an in-depth analysis of both the nature of the phenomenon and the ways in which it was addressed during the Soviet era, as demonstrated by this review of Stalinist biomedical and administrative-repressive responses to opium consumption in Gorno-Badakhshan. These appear to have a strong resonance with the multiple aspects of the ongoing 'drug war' in Central Asia characterized by the lack of adequate medical and social care, widespread violations of human rights, and repression at the hands of law-enforcement agencies.

Acknowledgements

The Central Asia Program, Institute for European, Russian, and Eurasian Studies, The Elliott School of International Affairs, George Washington University; Global Health Research Center of Central Asia (GHRCCA), Columbia University, New York, USA.

Notes

1. Located in the Pamirs region, Mountainous Badakhshan Autonomous Oblast (Gorno-Badakhshanskaia Avtonomnaia Oblast' or GBAO) was officially founded in January 1925 and made part of the Tajik Autonomous Soviet Socialist Republic; at that time it was referred to as AGBO. In numerous publications on GBAO, it is interchangeably referred to as the Pamir(s), 'the roof of the world', Gorno-Badakhshan and Soviet Badakhshan (as far as its Soviet history is concerned).
2. According to one estimate made in 1901 (Aknazarov 2005a), there were 683 households in Rushan, 512 in Shugnan and 219 in Vakhan and Ishkashim, with a total population of 13,796 people.
3. Such time would have come as early as in the 1920s, when all Cherkesov's wishes were implemented by the Bolsheviks to the degree that he could hardly imagine when writing his report.
4. RGVIA [The Russian State Archive of Military History], f. 1396, op. 2 dop., d. 2167, l. 99.
5. In pre-Soviet Central Asia, opium smoking was mainly prevalent in areas bordering (or otherwise closely connected due to commercial links) with China and Persia, with Turkmen people generally considered being most affected (Latypov 2008).
6. Unfortunately, Shergaziev himself (or Shergaziev's original source, the Party Archive of the Institute of History of the Communist Party at the Central Committee of the Communist Party of Uzbekistan, f. 58, op. 4, d. 344, l. 61) did not specify the date to which this estimate applies, but the title of his paper implies its relationship to the post-revolutionary period of 1920–9. Other archival records paint a similar picture in the Pamirs in the 1920s and provide a similar 'estimate' of 'up to 90%' of all financial means being spent on opium. In later publications by Tajik historians, who reproduced the same estimate and either referred to Shergaziev directly or to the Uzbek Communist Party Archive, there is some confusion in terms of the period to which this estimate applies. Iskandarov and Iusupov (1976) supply this account as a context for the 1906 prohibition; Odilbekova (1984) also suggests its relation to the pre-revolutionary Pamir; Nazarshoev (1970, 1982) insists that the estimate was given for the first years of Soviet rule in the Pamirs.
7. According to TsGA RT [The Central State Archive of the Republic of Tajikistan], f. 172, op. 1, d. 6, ll. 193–196, the hospital in Khorog had 20 beds in 1930, whereas the Rushan-based hospital had 10.
8. Tal'iants' surname is spelled as Tel'iants in most other publications.
9. TsGA RT, f. 10, op. 1, d. 289, ll. 27–28.
10. RGASPI [The Russian State Archive of Social and Political History], f. 62, op. 2, d. 1272, ll. 3–4; TsGA RT, f. 172, op. 1, d. 14, ll. 163–169.
11. See also TsGA RT, f. 172, op. 1, d. 32, l. 54. Tel'iants insists that this replacement resulted from the efforts of the local party organization in Gorno-Badakhshan. However, based on the activity report of the Tajik *Narkomzdrav* during the first six months of 1928, and particularly the findings of *Narkomzdrav*'s surveys in Kuliab, Kurgan-Tube and former Hissar regions, it seems that this step of removing unqualified medical personnel was part of the wider changes in *Narkomzdrav*'s policies towards 'peripheries'. See TsGA RT, f. 172, op. 1, d. 14, ll. 188–202.
12. However, Slavnin's estimate raises some questions. As some archival reports of the Tajik *Narkomzdrav* indicate, contrary to Paradoksov's publications, the denominator of 4640 (that is, the total number of residents in Rushan district) may need to be applied with regard to the number of opium addicts reported by Slavnin, thus further reducing the prevalence of opium addiction in Rushan in 1926 from 11.4% down to 7.3%. See TsGA RT, f. 172, op. 1, d. 38 t. 2, l. 382.
    In later publications by Tajik doctors and historians Slavnin's surname has nearly always been misspelled as either Slavin or even Slavina. Also, the issue of opium addiction as the main focus of Slavnin's survey in Rushan has disappeared from later works that cited his findings.
13. It is important to note that it is the *smoking* of opium that early Soviet authors emphasized and identified as '*narkomania*' in the Pamirs whereas the 'eating' of opium attracted almost no attention and did not seem to create serious tensions between the regime and the consumers.
14. TsGA RT, f. 10, op. 1, d. 290, l. 32; TsGA RT, f. 279, op. 2, d. 111, l. 15.
15. TsGA RT, f. 279, op. 3, d. 54, ll. 2–4ob, 12, 13.

16. The resolution of the Communist Party on the Pamirs issued in the same period also emphasized deficiencies in the struggle against opium smoking along the ‘treatment and prevention line’. See PAIPI TsK KP RT [The Party Archive of the Institute for Political Research of the Republic of Tajikistan Communist Party Central Committee], f. 3, op. 6, d. 61, l. 59.
17. PAIPI TsK KP RT, f. 3, op. 1, d. 62, l. 11; TsGA RT, f. 279, op. 4, d. 59, l. 1.
18. See also TsGA RT, f. 279, op. 4, d. 59, l. 3.
19. TsGA RT, f. 279, op. 7, d. 74, ll. 56–61; TsGA Tadzhikskoi SSR, f. 279, op. 5, d. 15, ll. 4–7 (in Radzhabov 1966).
20. The first Pamiri doctors, N. A. Kashkorova and A. O. Odinamamadov, graduated from the Tajik State Medical Institute in Stalinabad in summer 1954 and were posted in Gorno-Badakhshan.
21. TsGA RT, f. 279, op. 14, d. 178, ll. 1–28.
22. In the context of the opium war in Gorno-Badakhshan in the 1920s, where the police functioned as part of/under the administrative department of the local executive authorities, administrative struggle was often identical to law enforcement.
23. TsGA RT, f. 9, op. 1, d. 257, ll. 52–53.
    It should be noted that the initial ‘signs’ of the Soviet struggle against opium consumers in Gorno-Badakhshan appeared long before the 1925 First Pamir Congress of Soviets. Already in 1923 Shirinshoh Shotemur was writing to the Turkestan Central Executive Committee that opium users were not eligible to be elected into the Revolutionary Committees (Revkoms) in the Western Pamir (Nazarshoev 1970). In June 1925, four months before the Pamir Congress, the militia of Gorno-Badakhshan was praised by the Tajik ASSR Revkom for their struggle against drug smuggling and smoking of opium and cannabis (Imomyorbekov 2009). In June 1925, the *Krasnaia Niva* journal also published a celebratory article on the achievements of Soviet workers in the Pamirs and their struggle against opium smokers who were alien to the new regime (Gavriliuk and Iaroshenko 1987).
24. TsGA RT, f. 9, op. 1, d. 257, ll. 95, 95ob.
25. See also TsGA RT, f. 10, op. 1, d. 289, l. 27.
    The proposal to offer financial rewards to informants was made at the Presidium of the GBAO Executive Committee after reviewing the results of the administrative struggle against opium smoking achieved between April and August 1928. One of the findings of that review was a dramatic fall in drug seizures, as they decreased nearly four times between 1927 and 1928. In the next years, ‘the administrative department’ tended to ascribe the lack of seizures during some periods to its inability to deploy a wide network of secret collaborators because of the deficiency of funds. See GA GBAO [The State Archive of Gorno-Badakhshan Autonomous Oblast], f. 1, op. 1. d. 31, ll. 110, 111.
26. GA GBAO, f. 1, op. 1. d. 31, ll. 110, 111.
27. RGASPI, f. 62, op. 2, ch. II, d. 2308, ll. 1, 11, 12.
28. TsGA RT, f. 10, op. 1, d. 289, ll. 143, 144; TsGA RT, f. 10, op. 1, d. 290, l. 33.
29. GA GBAO, f. 1, op. 1. d. 31, ll. 110, 111 in A. Imomyorbekov, ‘Rol’ Organov Militsii GBAO v Ukreplenii Pravoporiadka i Obespechenii Obschestvennoi Bezopasnosti v Periodakh Obrazovaniia Tadzhikskoi SSR (1918–1930) i Gosudarstvennoi Nezavisimosti Respubliki Tadzhikistan (1991–2007).’ Unpublished manuscript.
30. TsGA RT, f. 10, op. 1, d. 289, l. 28. Apparently, the anti-drug sanctions could be also limited to short-term compulsory labour and did not always include the exile from border areas.
31. PAIPI TsK KP RT, f. 3, op. 1, d. 62, l. 11.
32. RGASPI, f. 17, op. 162, d. 10, ll. 65, 70, 71 (in Khaustov, Naumov, and Plotnikova 2003, 273–274); RGASPI, f. 62, op. 2, ch. II, d. 2308, ll. 1, 11, 12, 32.
33. RGASPI, f. 62, op. 2, ch. II, d. 2308, ll. 1, 11, 12, 49; RGASPI, f. 62, op. 2, d. 1504, ll. 2, 3, 9; TsGA RT, f. 10, op. 1, d. 290, l. 32. For an image of “Tajik Pamiri woman smoking opium” in 1928, see Lentz (1931), photograph between pp. 288 and 289; in addition, see http://rutube.ru/video/eec653341d855 34d620033b17cf0217e/ (Avtorskaia Programma Arkadiia Mamontova, ‘Spetsialnyi Korrespondent. Trafik’).
34. TsGA RT, f. 10, op. 1, d. 289, ll. 27, 143, 144. This goal was articulated by doctors only in 1932 (Tal’iants 1933), almost four years after it was spelt out by the militiamen. Physicians placed particular emphasis on keeping women and schoolchildren away from an ‘evil [drug] habit’, although these words remained words alone.
    The adoption of this goal also has clear implications for our interpretation of the writings by external groups visiting the region in the late 1920s and early 1930s, since they might have possibly seen only the superficial, visible part of the actual picture.
35. TsGA RT, f. 10, op. 1, d. 290, l. 33.

36. RGASPI, f. 62, op. 2, d. 1504, ll. 3, 6, 10; TsGA RT, f. 10, op. 1, d. 289, ll. 27, 28, 144; TsGA RT, f. 10, op. 1, d. 290, ll. 32, 33.
37. PAIPI TsK KP RT, f. 3, op. 1, d. 62, l. 11.
38. RGASPI, f. 62, op. 2, ch. II, d. 2308, ll. 48, 51, 52.
39. TsGA RT, f. 10, op. 1, d. 289, l. 27; TsGA RT, f. 10, op. 1, d. 290, ll. 32, 33. Concerns about the authority of the anti-opium-smoking society have been raised since the very moment it was proposed to set up that institution. In Shugnan volost', participants of the *Bespartiinaia Konferentsiia* believed that involving members of this society in the decision-making process of 'all sorts of Soviet and public organizations' on such vital issues as allocation and enlargement of land plots as well as disbursement of loans and benefits might help to raise the authority of the society and to recruit more members.
40. RGASPI, f. 62, op. 2, ch. II, d. 2308, l. 28; RGASPI, f. 17, op. 27, d. 14, ll. 166, 168. Note that (for known reasons) Nazarshoev (1970) claims that the major part of all credits was spent as intended, on purchasing live cattle, and not on narcotic drugs.
41. TsGA RT, f. 10, op. 1, d. 289, l. 27; RGASPI, f. 17, op. 27, d. 14, ll. 166, 167, 168.
42. RGASPI, f. 62, op. 2, ch. II, d. 2308, ll. 12, 28.
43. TsGA RT, f. 11, op. 14, d. 10, l. 115. I am very thankful to Botakoz Kassymbekova for sharing her TsGA RT records related to this issue with me.
    Another source that mentions opium smoking in Kurgan-Tube by settlers from the Pamirs is L. F. Paradoksov (1932, 1933).
44. APRF [The Archive of the President of the Russian Federation], f. 3, op. 58, d. 202, ll. 134–136 (in Khaustov, Naumov, and Plotnikova 2003, 517–518).
45. APRF, f. 3, op. 58, d. 202, ll. 134–136.
46. APRF, f. 3, op. 58, d. 202, ll. 134–136.
47. Paul Bergne (2007) writes that the Tajik–Afghan border was officially closed in 1936. In practice, however, control over the border remained very poor at least until late 1937, and crossing the Piandzh River from either side presented no challenge at all (other than that presented by the river itself). See A. A. Andreev to I. V. Stalin, 2 October 1937, RGASPI, f. 73, op. 2, d. 19, ll. 87–88 (in Kvashonkin et al. 1999, 377–379).
48. A. A. Andreev to I. V. Stalin, 2 October 1937. RGASPI, f. 73, op. 2, d. 19, ll. 87–88.
49. Operativnyi Prikaz Narodnogo Kommissara Vnutrennikh Del Soiuza SSR No. 00447 'Ob Operatsii po Repressirovaniiu Byvshikh Kulakov, Ugolovnikov i dr. Anti-Sovetskikh Elementov', 30 July 1937.
50. A. A. Andreev to I. V. Stalin, 2 October 1937. RGASPI, f. 73, op. 2, d. 19, ll. 87–88. For an account by one of the victims of these repressions, who provides a description of Andreev's visit to Tajikistan and subsequent arrests, see Nurmukhamedov 1988, 127–137.
51. According to one recent study (Zhirnov 2009) on the basis of materials from the Russian archives, Andrei Andreev initially began to use opiates in the 1940s in order to manage pain in one of his ears.
52. I am very thankful to the Tajik Ministry of Health and to the senior management of the Republican Clinical Psychiatric Hospital No. 1 in Rudaki District for granting me the permission to study these records.

References

Aknazarov, O., ed. 2005a. *Istoriia Gorno-Badakhshanskoi Avtonomnoi Oblasti*. Vol. I, Dushanbe: Paivand.

Aknazarov, O., ed. 2005b. *Istoriia Gorno-Badakhshanskoi Avtonomnoi Oblasti*. Vol. II, Dushanbe: Paivand.

Antsyferov, L. 1934. *Gashishizm v Srednei Azii*, 8–9. Tahskent: Prilozhenie k Zhurnalu Za Sotsialisticheskoe Zdravookhranenie Uzbekistana.

Averkiev, S. 1905a. "Vrachebnaia Pomosch Pamirskomy Naseleniiu." *Turkestanskie Vedomosti* 178: 934–935.

Averkiev, S. 1905b. "Vrachebnaia Pomosch Pamirskomy Naseleniiu." *Turkestanskie Vedomosti* 185: 977–978.

Averkiev, S. 1905c. "Vrachebnaia Pomosch Pamirskomy Naseleniiu." *Turkestanskie Vedomosti* 186: 985–986.

Bergne, P. 2007. *The Birth of Tajikistan: National Identity and the Origins of the Republic*. London: I.B. Tauris.

Bliss, F. 2006. *Social and Economic Change in the Pamirs (Gorno-Badakhshan, Tajikistan)*. Translated and edited by Nicola Pacult and Sonia Guss with the support of Tim Sharp. London and New York: Routlege.

Davliat'erov, D. 1974. "Razvitie Zdravookhraneniia na Pamire v Gody Zavversheniia Stroitel'stva Sotsializma (1946–1958 gg.)." In *Tadzhikistan v Bratskoi Sem'e Narodov SSSR*, edited by B. Iskandarov, K. Marsakov and L. Sechkina, 147–156. Dushanbe: Donish.
Gavriliuk, A., and V. Iaroshenko. 1987. *Pamir*. Moscow: Planeta.
Guliamov, M. 1963. "Predvaritel'nye Dannye o Techenii Nekotorykh Psikhicheskikh Zabolevanii v Usloviiakh Vysokogor'ia." *Zhurnal Nevropatologii i Psikhiatrii Imeni S. S. Korsakova* 63 (9): 1411–1413.
Guliamov, M. 1980. "Istoriia i Sovremennoe Sostoianie Bor'by s Narkomaniei v Tadzhikskoi SSR." *Zdravookhranenie Tadzhikistana* 3: 85–89.
Guliamov, M. 1987. "Dostizheniia i Perspektivy Razvitiia Psikhiatrii v Tadzhikistane. K 70-Letiiu Velikogo Oktiabria." *Zdravookhranenie Tadzhikistana* 4: 6–14.
Guliamov, M. 1988. "Gashishnaia Narkomaniia." *Zdravookhranenie Tadzhikistana* 2: 36–41.
Guliamov, M., and A. Pogosov. 1987. *Narkomaniia: Klinika, Diagnostika, Lechenie, Profilaktika*. Dushanbe: Irfon.
Gulomov, M., S. Sharofov, and M. Kleandrov. 1989. *Muborizai ziddi Nash'amandi va Zahrmandi*. Dushanbe: Irfon.
Guliamov, M., and A. Subbotin. 1972. "Psikhiatricheskaia Pomosch i Perspectivy ee Razvitiia v Tadzhikistane." *Zdravookhranenie Tadzhikistana* 6: 54–61.
Guliamov, M., and A. Subbotin. 1984. "Razvitie Psikhiatricheskoi Nauki i Praktiki." *Zdravookhranenie Tadzhikistana* 4: 17–23.
Imomyorbekov, A. 2009. "Iz Istorii Formirovaniia i Razvitiia Deiatel'nosti Tadzhikskoi Militsii na Pamire v Period s 1918 po 1945gg." *Izvestiia Akademii Nauk Respubliki Tadzhikistan, Otdeleniie Obschestvennykh Nauk* 2: 13–23.
Iskandarov, B., and Sh. Iusupov. 1976. "Russkie Vrachi na Pamire." *Izvestiia Akademii Nauk Tadzhikskoi SSR, Otdelenie Obschestvennykh Nauk* 3: 34–40.
Iunge, M., G. Bordiukov, and R. Binner. 2008. *Vertikal' Bol'shogo Terrora: Istoriia Operatsii po Prikazu NKVD No 00447*. Moscow: Novyi Khronograph.
Keshavjee, S. 1998. "Medicines and Transitions: The Political Economy of Health and Social Change in Post-Soviet Badakhshan, Tajikistan." PhD diss., Harvard University.
Khaustov, V., V. Naumov, and N. Plotnikova, eds. 2003. *Lubianka: Stalin i VCHK-GPU-OGPU-NKVD, Ianvar' 1922 – Dekabr' 1936*. Moscow: Izdatel'stvo 'Materik'.
Kholdarbekov, I. 1983. "Istoriia Zarozhdeniia i Sovremennoe Sostoianie Psikhiatricheskoi Pomoschi Naseleniiu GBAO." In *Aktual'nye Voprosy Psikhiatrii*, edited by Minkhodzh Guliamov, 22–24. Dushanbe: Ministerstvo Zdravookhraneniia Tadzhikskoi SSR.
Korovnikov, A. 1929. "Po Doline Vancha." *Meditsinskaia Mysl' Uzbekistana i Turkmenistana* 6-7: 59–68.
Kvashonkin, A., L. Kosheleva, L. Rogovaia, and O. Khlevniuk, eds. 1999. *Sovetskoe Rukovodstvo. Perepiska*, 1928–1941. Moscow: ROSSPEN.
Latypov, A. 2008. "Medicine, Culture and Empire: European Encounters with the Opium Consumer in Russian Central Asia, 1867–1917." MA diss., University College London.
Latypov, A. 2010. "Healers and Psychiatrists: The Transformation of Mental Health Care in Tajikistan." *Transcultural Psychiatry* 47 (3): 419–451.
Latypov, A. 2011a. "The Administration of Addiction: The Politics of Medicine and Opiate Use in Soviet Tajikistan, 1924–1958." PhD diss., University College London.
Latypov, A. 2011b. "The Soviet Doctor and the Treatment of Drug Addiction: A Difficult and Most Ungracious Task." *Harm Reduction Journal* 8 (32). doi:10.1186/1477-7517-8-32.
Latypov, A. 2012. *On the Road to 'H': Narcotic Drugs in Soviet Central Asia*. Washington, DC: The George Washington University, The Elliott School of International Affairs, Central Asia Program.
Lentz, W. 1931. *Auf dem Dach der Welt. Mit Phonograph und Kamera bei vergessenen Völkern des Pamir*. Berlin: Deutsche Buch-Gemeinschaft.
Luknitsky, P. 1954. *Soviet Tajikistan*. Moscow: Foreign Languages Publishing House.
Luknitskii, P. 1955. *Puteshestviia po Pamiru*. Moscow: Izdatel'stvo TsK VLKSM 'Molodaia Gvardiia.
Mirzobekov, M. 1974. "Istoriia Razvitiia Zdravookhraneniia Sovetskogo Pamira." *Zdravookhranenie Tadzhikistana* 3: 5–9.
Motylev, Ia. 1977. *Dokumenty Svidetel'stvuiut: Kratkii Ocherk Istorii Tadzhikskoi Militsii*. Dushanbe: Irfon.
Nurmukhamedov, M. 1988. "Tak Bylo...Iz Vospominanii." *Pamir* 11: 127–137.
Nazarshoev, M. 1970. *Partiinaia Organizatsiia Pamira v Bor'be za Sotsializm i Kommunizm*, 1918–1968. Dushanbe: Irfon.

Nazarshoev, M. 1982. *Istoricheskii Opyt KPSS po Rukovodstvu Sotsialisticheskim Stroitel'stvom v Gorno-Badakhshanskoi Avtonomnoi Oblasti Tadzhikskoi SSR*, 1917–1941. Dushanbe: Donish.

Odilbekova, R. 1984. "Kul'tura Zapadnogo Pamira v Kontse XIX – Nachale XX v." In *Pamirovedenie.* Vol. II, edited by M. S. Asimov, 7–22. Dushanbe: Donish.

Olufsen, O. 1904. *Through the Unknown Pamirs: The Second Danish Pamir Expedition*, 1898–99. London: William Heinemann.

Ostrovsky, A. 1955. "Dar Bobati Zarari Tamokukashi." *Badakhshoni Soveti* 60 (2028): 4.

Paradoksov, L. 1932. "Materialy k Izucheniiu Zabolevaemosti Korennogo Naseleniia Tadzhikistana." *Za Sotsialisticheskoe Zdravookhranenie Uzbekistana* 4: 67–70.

Paradoksov, L. 1933. "Nekotorye Dannye ob Istorii Zdravookhraneniia i Zabolevaemosti Naseleniia Tadzhikistana." *Zdravookhranenie Tadzhikistana* 1: 18–25.

Propaschikh. 1903. "Upotreblenie Opiia v Vakhane, Shugnane i Rushane." *Turkestanskie Vedomosti* 43: 263–264.

Radzhabov, Z., ed. 1966. *Iz Istorii Kul'turnogo Stroitel'stva v Tadzhikistane v*, 1924–1941gg. Vol. I. Dushanbe: Irfon.

Rakhimov, P. 1955. "Khizmatrasonii Tibbi ba Aholi Behtar Karda Shavad." *Badakhshoni Soveti* 60 (2028): 2.

Rayner, O., trans. 1925. *The Criminal Code of the Russian Socialist Federative Soviet Republic.* London: H. M. Stationery Office.

Shansky, L. 1954. "Razvitie Zdravookhraneniia na Pamire." *Zdravookhranenie Tadzhikistana* 2: 9–11.

Shergaziev, M. 1959. "Iz Istorii Bor'by Kommunisticheskoi Partii za Vostanovlenie i Razvitie Ekonomiki i Kul'tury GBAO (1920–1929gg.)." In *Ocherki po Istorii Tadzhikistana.* Vol. II, edited by A. A. Benediktov, 73–90. Stalinabad: Stalinabadskii Gosudarstvennyi Pedagogicheskii Institut im. T. T. Shevchenko.

Tal'iants, N. 1933. "Zdravookhranenie v Avt. Gorno-Badakhshanskoi Oblasti." *Zdravookhranenie Tadzhikistana* 1: 79–86.

Teliiants, N. 1974. "Rasskazyvaiut Veterany Zdravookhraneniia." *Zdravookhranenie Tadzhikistana* 5: 48–50.

Tkhostova, V. 1988. "Fel'dsher-Revoliutsioner." *Zdravookhranenie Tadzhikistana* 3: 92–93. http://kommersant.ru/doc/1164102.

Zhirnov, E. 2009. "Progressiruiuschee Istoschenie Nervnoi Sistemy." *Kommersant Vlast* 19 (823).

Mentally ill or chosen by spirits? 'Shamanic illness' and the revival of Kazakh traditional medicine in post-Soviet Kazakhstan

Danuta Penkala-Gawęcka

Department of Ethnology and Cultural Anthropology, Adam Mickiewicz University, Poznań, Poland

This article discusses spiritual healing in post-Soviet Kazakhstan with reference to changing discourses about 'shamanic illness': a condition that afflicts the future healer. What had traditionally been identified as the call of spirits was seized in the Soviet period by biomedical discourse which ascribed those symptoms to mental illness. Whereas this attitude also influenced popular understandings of 'shamanic illness' at the time, traditional ideas have been gradually restored in the context of the political and social changes of the 1990s. Biomedical discourse on 'shamanic illness' has also undergone significant changes. I argue that this was induced by multiple interconnected factors, among which are the reappraisal and support of the government for Kazakh 'folk' medicine as a part of the national heritage, and a favourable attitude to local, traditional forms of religiosity. This allowed for collaboration between doctors and healers in the context of institutionalization of traditional medicine. Alongside these influences the strength of the tradition of remembering the spirits of ancestors prompted the re-establishment of this core experience in the process of becoming a healer: the call of spirits.

Many researchers working in Central Asia, especially those interested in the 'revival' of Islam and broader questions of religious life, have noticed a surge of medical pluralism in the post-Soviet period. There is an apparent multiplicity of healing methods that have developed since the collapse of the Soviet Union, and their relations with biomedicine are shaped by complex economic, social and political factors. This phenomenon is, however, understudied apart from a few anthropological works (Hohmann 2007, 2010b; Penkala-Gawecka 2002). More attention has been paid to spiritual healing, that is, healing with the help of spirits,[1] which has been discussed mainly in the context of 'everyday Islam' as a part of what is locally perceived as 'Muslimness' (Kehl-Bodrogi 2008; Privratsky 2001; Rasanayagam 2006). Some researchers take other perspectives on this kind of healing, addressing the issues of its legitimization (Pelkmans 2005) or competition of healers in the market (Bellér-Hann 2001).

This article explores spiritual healing in the context of the vast field of medical pluralism in Kazakhstan.[2] The changed political and economic circumstances in post-Soviet Central Asia influenced the efflorescence of spiritual healing which draws heavily on traditional beliefs and practices. I focus on a particular aspect – the so called 'shamanic illness' – which was traditionally perceived as a sign of predestination and a preliminary stage on the way to becoming a shaman. My purpose is to show changing perceptions of its symptoms that have led to a contemporary revalidation of its original meaning in popular and partly in biomedical discourses.

I argued that the support of the government for Kazakh 'folk' medicine, treated as a part of national heritage, and nation-building policy significantly contributed to the rehabilitation of spiritual healing. In addition, the favourable official attitude to local forms of 'Muslimness' and the lively tradition of remembering the spirits of ancestors, helped to recover the traditional discourse on 'shamanic illness'. Nevertheless, other factors should also be taken into account, including the weak public health-care system that influenced the process of the institutionalization of traditional medicine, enabling close contacts between physicians and healers.

The text is based on in-depth fieldwork that I carried out in Kazakhstan during my five-year stay there between 1995 and 2000, mainly in Almaty and its vicinity. The main focus of my studies was complementary medicine set in its wider political and socio-economic context, as well as complementary practitioners – healers and doctors – and their patients. I collected ethnographic material in the course of many talks with spiritual healers, including shamans, and during observations of their séances in different settings.

Traditional Kazakh shamans and 'shamanic illness'

The healing practices of shamans were only a part of Kazakh medical traditions, which comprised various therapies practised by a range of specialists, like bone-setters (*sınıqshı*), herbalists (*däriger*) or folk surgeons (*otashı*) who performed bloodletting and minor operations. In addition, methods used by *täwips* (from Arabic: *tabib*) consisted of elements of Arabic-Persian-Tajik 'great medical tradition' (*Unani*) based on written transmission, which was, however, more popular in other parts of Central Asia (Penkala-Gawęcka 2009; Sharmanov and Atchabarov 1978).

Kazakh spiritual healing was practised mainly by shamans (*baqsı*) whose supernatural powers, purportedly enabled them to mediate between spirits and the human world. Veneration of ancestor spirits (*arūaq*) was at the core of Kazakh spirituality and shaped their shamanic practices. The *baqsı*, usually a man,[3] used various techniques aimed at expelling evil spirits with the assistance of his helping spirits (Basilov 1992, 146–154).

In addition to shamans, mullahs, *ishans* (Sufi shaykhs) and itinerant dervishes (*dūana*) depended on contacts with the supernatural world in their healing. They recited verses from the Qur'an and prepared amulets (*tumar*) against harmful spirits and the evil eye. Like shamans, they were known for their skills in curing mental disorders through exorcisms.[4] The process of Islamization of the Kazakh shamanic performances was already well advanced in the late nineteenth and early twentieth centuries. Besides ancestral spirits they invoked Muslim saints and Allah, and included prayers from the Qur'an in their healing. The shamanic séance was called *oyın* (play) or *zikir* (from Arabic *dhikr*) – the last term used for ecstatic performances in Sufi brotherhoods. As DeWeese (1994, 51, 54) points out, these facts may be taken not only as the evidence of Islamization of the earlier local beliefs and practices, but also as indigenization of Islam which assimilated those traditions and granted them reaffirmation.

A traditional way of becoming a shaman in Central Asia involved a kind of rite of passage which started with an episode of 'shamanic illness',[5] often described in ethnographic reports. It included strange dreams and visions, unusual behaviours and persistent suffering of the afflicted. It should be stressed that those symptoms were differentiated from madness or other mental disorders that, in local perceptions, required the intervention of the healer. The initiation experiences usually induced separation of an afflicted individual from the community and were often accompanied by serious physical ailments like loss of sight or paralysis.

That particular condition was easily recognizable in the past. Shamanic abilities could be transmitted from a former shaman to someone who belonged to the next generation or to the generation of their grandchildren. However, the call of spirits was crucial and a person chosen by the ancestor spirits (*arūaq*) was obliged to accept their gift. When after the shaman's death one of his descendants fell seriously ill, it was taken as a sign given by the spirits (Basilov 1992, 128–129; Toleubaev 1997), clear both to the future *baqsı* and to all members of the community. Put in another way, within the traditional frame just getting ill with specific symptoms elicited recognition of this suffering as the call of spirits and entering the liminal phase of the rite of passage. The process to follow could last quite a long time and during that stage a candidate was taught and tried by spirits. The change of status was marked then by a blessing received from spirits and sometimes from an older, experienced shaman or a respected religious man.

Attitudes to shamans and other traditional healers during Russian and Soviet times

It is significant that many reports of the travellers and ethnographers of the late eighteenth and the nineteenth centuries dealt with 'shamanism' in Central Asia whereas not many sources referred to other methods of healing (Basilov 1992, 30–39). This fixation on shamanic rituals was noted by the researchers who criticize the tendency to neglect other important or even more central aspects of religious life of the local peoples like domestic cults and remembering dead ancestors in particular (Bellér-Hann 2001; DeWeese 1994; Kehl-Bodrogi 2008).

It is worth noting that such an approach coincided with the Russian imperial policies of those times. The Kazakh shaman's figure epitomized the wildness and backwardness of the native population. His healing methods were usually presented as 'tricks', ineffective and harmful (Afanas'eva 2008, 132–133). If not seen as sly deceivers, shamans were often described as individuals with serious mental disorders. That view was present in both biomedical approach and ethnographic accounts of those times and also persisted during the Soviet era (see, for example Alimkhanov 1978; for a critical discussion see Basilov [1992, 106–110]).[6] In Michaels' opinion: 'This scholarship became the foundation for discrediting traditional medical practices, and for placing a monopoly of medical authority in biomedical practitioners' hands' (2003, 9). However, the attitude to other traditional forms of treatment was more ambivalent. Some doctors acknowledged that particular therapies might be effective and sometimes even better than methods of Russian medicine.[7] It is clear, anyway, that critical assessments of shamans' and mullahs' healing practices as well as of other habits of the local peoples constituted a ground for the Russian 'civilizing mission' (Afanas'eva 2008, 133; Hohmann 2010a; Michaels 2003, 35).[8]

The Soviet period brought about attempts to modernize the Central Asian region. Despite revolutionary slogans, those efforts, as many researchers note (for example, Michaels 2003; Roy 2000), were based on the ideological foundations laid during the Russian colonial period. Referring to traditional healing, Privratsky states: 'Russian scholarship treated the shaman as an obsolescent survivor of the nomadic cultural phase and thus encouraged the Soviet attack on the old healing arts' (2004, 570). Spiritual healers, together with mullahs, were treated as particularly harmful, although Soviet propaganda also presented other traditional medical practices as ineffective and even dangerous. However, despite severe persecutions of mullahs and shamans during the first decades of the new regime, traditional healing was not abandoned. Healers continued to work underground and then, towards the end of the Soviet Union, more and more openly. Michaels, using archival material and a survey conducted in Southern Kazakhstan, concludes that 'shamans and mullahs continued to serve the population, albeit in secret, throughout the Soviet era' (2003, 67). Indeed, my informants from Almaty often told me that it had been possible during Soviet times to find, if need be, a good, strong shaman through informal links.

Baqsı and other spiritual healers in the context of medical pluralism in post-Soviet Kazakhstan

I studied the path of the healer in the context of medical pluralism and the role of complementary medicine in post-Soviet Kazakhstan. The array of non-biomedical methods and techniques available to the people was very wide, from the local medical traditions of various ethnic groups, through Chinese, Tibetan and Indian 'great medical traditions', to many new or relatively new therapies borrowed from Russia, Ukraine and the West. I was interested in the reasons for the growing interest in such methods and for the official approval that, as I believe, justifies the use of the term complementary medicine in this context.

Whereas this stance diverges from the previous Soviet policy, it should be remembered that it was already in the 1970s–80s, in the period of 'late socialism' and *perestroika*, that some kinds of non-biomedical therapies were approved.[9] In particular, a new category of healers called *ekstrasensy*, whose treatment was based on the concept of bio-energy, became increasingly popular across the Soviet Union. These phenomena show that the relations between biomedicine and alternative/complementary medicine in the Soviet and post-Soviet conditions should not be viewed as so strikingly different. It could be reasonably argued that among the most important reasons for the rise in interest in non-biomedical healing in the last decades of the Soviet Union was the crisis of legitimacy, or even 'delegitimation' (Aronson 2007) of professional medicine, connected with the failing Soviet economy. The break-up of the Soviet Union exposed the weakness of the health-care system and brought about its further, dramatic deterioration in post-Soviet states. I agree with Brown and Rusinova (2002) and Aronson (2007) who wrote about the rejection of professional medicine in contemporary Russia, that the turn to alternative medicine is due mainly to the declining public trust in health-care institutions. However, other factors influencing the public interest and official attitude to non-biomedical treatments should also be taken into account.

The policy of Kazakhstan's government towards complementary medicine can be described as generally positive or even supportive. Some of its branches, labelled officially as 'traditional medicine' (for example, Chinese and Korean acupuncture, hirudotherapy [use of leeches] and homeopathy) have been incorporated into the health-care system; they are taught at several medical universities and at the Almaty Institute for the Advancement of Physicians. The other sector, which was defined as 'folk medicine', includes such diverse methods and practices as spiritual healing, herbalism, bone-setting and 'bio-energy therapy'. They have also been accepted, although their position seems less stable.

It is apparent that the collapse of the health-care system in the newly independent Republic of Kazakhstan influenced considerably the stance of the authorities who promoted non-biomedical methods and remedies as inexpensive and easily available. Yet the other important reasons for the governmental acceptance of Kazakh medical traditions were closely connected with the nation-building policy. What had earlier been viewed as 'survivals' that would disappear with the process of modernization became an important part of Kazakh cultural heritage. The various acts of Parliament 'About the Health of the Nation of the Republic of Kazakhstan' (of 1992, 1997 and 2003) stressed the role of folk medicine as a valuable complement to the health-care system. This approach was in keeping with the overall revalidation of the traditions of the titular nation, important for the legitimization of the new state. Similar processes were observed in other post-Soviet Central Asian countries, such as Uzbekistan (Hohmann 2007; Kehl-Bodrogi 2008) or Kyrgyzstan.

At the same time the Ministry of Health of the Republic of Kazakhstan attempted to control and regulate the free market of healers, and to accredit their practices with reference to approved standards. The Republican Centre of Eastern and Contemporary Medicine in Almaty, founded in 1990 as the Centre of Folk Medicine, was entrusted with the task of training and licensing the healers. I will present these activities and the relations between biomedicine and spiritual healing in more detail in the last section of this article.

There are several categories of healers in Kazakhstan who appeal to the supernatural in their practice. First, shamans (Kaz. *baqsı,* Uyg. *bakhshı*) whose power is considered extraordinary and rare. Second, there are 'ordinary' spiritual healers (*täwip*) who usually combine spiritual healing with divination. Both categories resort to prayers from the Qur'an and supplications to Allah and saints in their practice. Mullahs (*molda*) also practise healing through the use of prayers.

Privratsky (2001, 194–195), in his book on the religious life of Kazakhs from the southern part of the country, proposed similar categorization of the Kazakh healers, but he only made brief references to the 'living Kazak shamans' and in most cases expressed a doubt over their shamanic identities. However, I met a few healers who called themselves *baqsı* and were recognized as shamans in the community; other researchers also mention shamans whom they approached during fieldwork in Kazakhstan (Bellér-Hann 2001, 2004; Grzywacz 2010; Jessa 2006a). I believe Privratsky's scepticism springs from his tendency to search for the 'authentic' *baqsı*. The Islamization of shamanic practices makes him call them 'faint images of archaic practice vaguely understood by Kazak healers themselves' (Privratsky 2001, 227). Here I adopt a local perspective on who is recognized as a *baqsı* and, on this basis, I cannot deny their presence among spiritual healers.

Shamans are thought to have special abilities and great powers thanks to the help of many powerful spirits. They have privileged connections with the spirit world; in the words of one of my informants 'they act as a bridge between earth and heaven'. Shamans may also have the gift of clairvoyance. Moreover, some characteristics of their séances such as trance states make them exceptional.

The 'ordinary' healers (*täwip*) are very popular – people ask them for help especially if they suspect that their health problems or misfortune have been caused by the evil eye (Kaz. *köz tiyū*; Rus. *sglaz*) or witchcraft. They search for a renowned *baqsı* in the case of serious and persistent troubles, especially if they are attributed to the influence of evil spirits (*jın*) or the so-called *porcha* (Rus.), particularly harmful black magic.

The practices of spiritual healers generally follow traditional patterns. They have traditional utensils for expelling the evil spirits: the whip (*qamshı*) and the knife (*pıshaq*). Those who practise divination use 41 stones or beans (*qumalaq*) for that purpose. In addition, the Qur'an and the rosary (*täspi*), signs of the Muslim identity of healers, form part of their equipment. Yet they borrow and assimilate some other methods and attributes, most eagerly those characteristic of *ekstrasensy*, like healing with 'bio-currents'. Hybridization is also seen in the 'pantheon of spirits' of contemporary healers who sometimes add to their helping spirits the saints and gods of other religions and even heroes of popular culture. (For similar examples on Buryat shamans see Humphrey [1999]). Despite a lack of sufficient data, it may be supposed that in more remote areas of the country hybridization of spiritual healing is not so marked. Healers in the city have a diverse clientele and they recognize that enrichment of the methods used may win them more popularity.

As I observed, spiritual healing based on belief in the world of spirits and their assistance in healing was popular in the Almaty of the 1990s among Kazakhs and other Turkic groups like Uyghurs or Tatars. Moreover, the patients of such healers were sometimes people of diverse ethnic origin, including Russians, Ukrainians or Germans.

'Shamanic illness' as the core experience in the making of a contemporary spiritual healer

Although the term 'shamanic illness' is a concept favoured by researchers, perhaps the more suitable term would be the 'call of spirits', more commonly recognized by people on the ground. However, because of the long tradition of the use of the former term in scholarly literature, I preserve it and apply it here also to other spiritual healers whose initiation exhibits very similar traits to those of the shaman.

As I already mentioned, despite Soviet attempts to eradicate traditional Kazakh medicine, some healing rituals, including shamanic practices, continued. Nevertheless, a long period of militant atheism brought about a considerable disruption to the healing traditions, especially in the cities. With the hegemony of biomedicine and its discourse, the traditional meaning of the symptoms of 'shamanic illness' was generally forgotten. Signs that had been earlier identified by the people as the 'call of spirits' were attributed by medical doctors to mental disturbances. In other words, what had been previously connected with the realm of the supernatural was seized by biomedical discourse and classified as mental illness. This scientific discourse, which influenced a popular attitude, established the practice that in the case of such unusual symptoms doctors – if they could not find any organic disease – diagnosed the sufferer as mentally impaired.

However, since the beginning of the 1990s, when healers started to practise openly, the traditional notions of 'shamanic illness' have been gradually revived.

I heard stories from many practitioners about their path to becoming a healer which revealed the same general pattern. Their sufferings started suddenly, sometimes provoked by a traumatic event or by a visit to *mazar* – a place where a saint or ancestors are buried. The afflicted individuals described their anxiety and distress, frightening visions and dreams in which they usually saw old, bearded men clothed in white. They also experienced physical symptoms of illness, often severe, and doctors could not help them. Because of those disturbances and strange behaviour, such as sudden attacks of panic and hearing voices, their relatives as well as doctors suspected mental illness and such persons often underwent psychiatric treatment, to no avail. When, at last, somebody advised them to visit a healer, their sufferings became intelligible. It was made clear by the spiritual specialist that the sufferer was someone chosen by spirits, and that strange dreams and visions were in fact revelations (*ayan*)[10] of their departed ancestors' will. They wanted to pass the healing gift (*darın*) to their descendant who should accept this and become a healer since the only way to recover was to comply with the spirits' demand. Otherwise, not only would the disobedient person be severely punished, but her/his close relatives might suffer and even die as well. Narratives of the healers reported widely on the terrible pain and suffering they had experienced until they accepted the 'call of spirits'. Those 'initiation stories' were strikingly similar, although healers differed in age, sex, ethnic origin (Kazakhs, Uyghurs, Uzbeks, Tatars), social background and education.[11]

I will give a few examples. Bayan, a Kazakh woman from a poor family living in a small village near Turkistan, had been continually affected by the evil eye since her early childhood, and every time a mullah helped her with recitation of the Qur'an. When Bayan's brother died, near the end of the 1980s, she visited the mausoleum of a famous Central Asian saint, Ahmad Yasawi, in Turkistan. A pious woman who recited prayers near the tomb told her that she should start to heal people, otherwise her close relatives would die prematurely. Bayan was frightened. However, she did not follow that advice, even though old men whom she saw in her dreams demanded that she accepted their gift. It was only after a series of accidents and deaths of some other members of her family that she decided to embrace the path of the healer. I also talked to Katya, a 50-year-old Kazakh historian from Almaty whose abilities were uncovered by Dilya, a healer and clairvoyant from the Centre of Eastern and Contemporary Medicine. Katya was afraid herself that she was mentally ill and her husband confirmed her in that belief. However, several visits to the Centre completely changed her view and she decided to quit her job and start to apprentice to Dilya.[12] It should be noted that apprenticeship also includes Islamic spiritual guidance of a neophyte.

Yet another Kazakh woman-healer and physician in her mid-50s, Tamara from Almaty, told me about her experience. At the beginning of the 1990s she developed strange symptoms – she had breathing difficulties at night and saw in her dreams a row of old men in white, repeating: 'You have to heal people.' Tamara did not understand that, and being afraid of having mental illness, went to a psychiatrist. However, her fears were not confirmed by the doctors nor were suppositions about a somatic illness. Then she met an acquaintance who had already begun working as a healer and they visited the Centre of Folk Medicine. After completing several courses of acupuncture, massage, astrology and learning the methods of Kazakh folk medicine, Tamara decided to combine them with biomedicine and started to work at the Centre. It is interesting in her case that although her path was more characteristic of urban eclectic practitioners, she received a traditional kind of blessing (*bata*: blessing for a new path, which was ritually given by a shaman) from a renowned, charismatic healer Umut apa (Mother Hope) who led a 'healing commune' near Pavlodar in Northern Kazakhstan.

An illustrative example is the case of an Uyghur *bakhshı*, Rakhilyam, living near Almaty, a woman in her early 50s then. As she told me, she had had such illness episodes twice. For the first time she was partially paralyzed, had convulsions and heard voices; sometimes a grimace suddenly twisted her face and she shouted involuntarily. She visited different medical specialists with no results. At last she was directed to a psychiatric clinic, but after a short stay there her sister took her to an old Uyghur shaman from the vicinity of Almaty. The shaman helped her, but – as Rakhilyam maintained – he did not reveal the truth about her abilities, because then, at the end of the 1980s, he was still afraid to talk about it. But when she visited the same shaman some years later complaining of strange symptoms again, he explained the meaning of her experiences. He revealed to Rakhilyam that she had 'shaman's blood': the shamanic gift offered by her ancestor spirits, which she was obliged to accept. When she decided to embrace the path of the shaman, she recovered entirely.

While in the past the call of spirits usually occurred in the period of adolescence, currently it often strikes a person of middle age who lived many years unaware of her/his potential. It is not surprising, if we consider the disruption to shamanic traditions. However, in the case of Mahira, Rakhilyam's daughter, the traditional pattern of an early revelation was observed. She had been offered the shamanic and clairvoyance gift when she was only 17, but since she did not feel ready, the spirits waited until her middle 20s. This motif of postponement, waiting until the future shaman feels prepared for her/his duties, is well known from the sources on shamanism in Central Asia. (See Goršunova [2000, 192–194] on a shaman-woman Khadicha from Osh region, Kyrgyzstan).

Some other cases of 'shamanic illness' experienced by present-day Kazakh healers are described by Grzywacz (2010, 26–28). Kehl-Bodrogi, who did insightful research into Khorezm healers (2008, 201–220), notices the importance of 'initiatory illness' and dream revelations. She points out: 'Although the "illness-pattern" in the case of healing is not exclusive to Central Asia and Siberia, in that context it does appear to be a particular cultural imperative, as the Khorezmian case also illustrates' (Kehl-Bodrogi 2008, 215–216).

The strength of the phenomenon of the call of spirits in contemporary Central Asia needs careful consideration. It cannot simply be attributed to the 'revival of tradition'. What seems particularly interesting here is the fact that 'shamanic illness' appears as a most immutable element of the local healing traditions. I think that this may be explained primarily by the importance of commemorating the spirits of ancestors, thoroughly discussed by Privratsky (2001). Noticeably, beliefs concerning the close ties between the living and the dead, and the influence of the latter on the lives of their descendants continued during Soviet times as did domestic rituals such as 'emitting of the smell' (of hot oil) for the ancestral spirits (Jessa 2006a, 363; Privratsky 2001, 128–133) which show great similarity across Central Asia (Kehl-Bodrogi 2008, 126–127). It is just these beliefs that underlie 'shamanic illness'. An important factor is that the 'call of spirits' appears crucial for the legitimization of healers, which I will discuss in the next section.

Such illness is a prerequisite for becoming a spiritual healer, but the role of training under a master seems to be quite important today. I observed several of Rakhilyam's healing séances and some of them revealed potential healers among the patients. In one case a *bakhshi* explained to her patient, a young Uyghur girl named Elmira, that her ailment was caused by the evil eye, which had already affected the girl in childhood. The girl was a 'spiritual person' (that is, someone with close connections with spirits), thus she was particularly vulnerable. The main point of the ritual was to purify Elmira. Next, the shaman explained that the spirits had offered two gifts to Elmira. First, the ability to heal people with prayers; second, the help of particular spirits who would come to her in the shape of birds. The girl seemed shocked by that revelation. Rakhilyam tried to convince her patient to obey the spirits' will, telling her that otherwise she would not recover. Rakhilyam also spotted future healers during other séances. An important part of the procedure of revealing candidates was pointing to the ancestors: shamans or other spiritual healers, or mullahs. Usually a person seems not to remember such predecessors and it is the experienced healer who makes her/him recall that. Being lineal kin of a 'spiritual person' definitely reinforces the claims of future practitioners, although it is the ancestor spirits who are believed to appoint someone among their living descendants. This follows the traditional pattern of the healer's legitimacy.

Similar examples of identification of future healers by the experienced ones are given by the researchers working in Central Asia (Bellér-Hann 2001, 79; Goršunova 2000, 201). According to Kehl-Bodrogi, a shared dream in which the future master and apprentice are 'shown' to each other is the precondition for the establishment of apprenticeship in healing in Khorezm (2008, 219). Such cases were also reported by some of my Kazakh informants, but rather with reference to the further development of healers.[13]

It was often stressed that in Central Asia, apprenticeship did not have an important place in the career of the shaman (Basilov 1992, 119–121; Toleubaev 1997, 199). However, in post-Soviet Kazakhstan, experienced senior healers play a crucial role in appointing and giving legitimacy to spiritual healers. Their authority revives and legitimizes the traditional meaning of strange symptoms and sufferings. It is the healer's diagnosis, presented as an expression of ancestor spirits' will, that starts a candidate's initiation and it is the healer's duty to make a person chosen by spirits accept the call as well as to assist her/him in this way. The relations between the master and the neophyte can be described as apprenticeship, although the actors themselves tend to belittle these ties and stress the main role of spirits in the paths of a healer (cf. Bellér-Hann 2001, 88–89).

An interesting phenomenon is the visible dominance of female healers, both in Kazakhstan and in other parts of Central Asia. In the case of the Kazakhs, it is justified to call this a gender shift, as previously the Kazakh shamans were mostly male. However, there are also men among contemporary spiritual (and other) healers, albeit in a minority.[14] The researchers tend to explain the feminization of healing by the diminishing prestige of these practices. It is suggested that women, as the most marginalized, took over what was abandoned by the men. According to a different view, the 'domestication' of shamanic practices during the Soviet times greatly contributed to this shift (for the discussion see Kehl-Bodrogi [2008, 198–199]). While the domestication argument seems reasonable and accords with the evidence of the significance of domestic rituals, performed by women, to religious continuity, I would not agree with the marginalization thesis. As my research indicates, healing can be the source of quite a good income, and there is an intense rivalry among the healers in this lucrative market (cf. Bellér-Hann 2001, 96). I would rather connect the interest of women in healing with their increasing agency. Some of the woman-healers whom I met achieved a high position, overtaking men in their families, and gained the respect of their community. Even if they were not all so successful, entering the 'healing profession' not only gave them some income, but also liberated them, at least partly, from other social obligations and familial relationships of dependence.

Local healing traditions in Kazakhstan have been strengthened by their close connections with Islamic religiosity. I wish to point out that spiritual healing, together with pilgrimages to sacred places or wearing amulets, is locally perceived in Kazakhstan and other parts of Central Asia as a truly Muslim practice. Many authors concur that it is an important component of what is called 'Muslimness' in the region (Grzywacz 2010; Kehl-Bodrogi 2008; Privratsky 2001; Rasanayagam 2006). This term, as Kehl-Bodrogi puts it, 'describes religion as it is lived rather than as it is defined by the theologians'. (2008, 84). I would add that there was evidence from Kazakhstan about some informal Islamic organizations, like Aq jol ('Pure Way'), established around 1997, whose main purpose was the revitalization of Muslim religiosity at the grass-roots level. It is significant that at the core of their activities were group séances of ritual purification and healing performed by charismatic spiritual leaders-healers. During Aq jol meetings, experienced healers revealed the potential healers with special abilities; they also organized collective pilgrimages to *mazar*s (Jessa 2006a, 2006b). In that way they actively contributed to the spread of ideas about the intercession of ancestor spirits in healing, as well as to the return to the previous communal character of the healing séances.

I can only briefly touch upon the complex issue of the 'official' Islamic discourse on local 'Muslimness', including spiritual healing. Most of the scholarship on Central Asian Islam denies a simplistic dichotomy of 'official' and 'unofficial' or 'popular' Islam. Nevertheless, researchers (Jessa 2006b; Omelicheva 2011) attest to the shift in the meaning of 'unofficial' Islam in the discourse of the governing regimes, the term 'now deployed in relation to the alleged threat of religious "extremism" and "fundamentalism"' (Omelicheva 2011, 245). Although the attitude of the Muslim Spiritual Directorate of Kazakhstan (*muftiyat*) towards 'popular' expressions of Islam is generally critical, the stance of the government to what is officially now called 'traditional' Islam may be characterized as positive, since it has been appropriated as closely associated with Kazakh ethnic and cultural identity. However, Omelicheva gives a detailed description of the on-going 'securitization' of Islam in Kazakhstan 'under the guise of combating terrorism and religious extremism' (2011, 251). This process may influence the attitude of the government to some local expressions of Muslim religiosity, and the criminalization of Aq jol in 2009 can serve as evidence of such changes.

Finally, the diagnosis that refers to the traditional idea of the 'call of spirits' instead of the label 'mentally ill' has important social consequences. Such a person is given credentials to become a healer, not sent to a psychiatrist. Moreover, spiritual healers themselves are treated as specialists who can help people with mental disorders. The acceptance of traditional illness etiologies (the evil eye, black magic, punishment by spirits, and so on) enhances the popularity of spiritual healers, especially in the case of chronic disturbances that are difficult to explain in biomedical terms. Kassymbekova (2003) writes about turning to spiritual healers in Southern Kazakhstan and Kyrgyzstan when mental illness occurs: a common practice reinforced by a lack of trust in mental-health facilities. According to the psychiatrists from Kyrgyzstan, from the local Kyrgyz point of view, 'an initial psychotic episode is usually considered a "spiritual emergence" and a patient generally has to visit a number of traditional healers before a psychiatrist takes care of him or her' (Molchanova et al. 2008, 68). Molchanova and Aĭtpaeva (2008) maintain that the trust in folk healers who offer their help to people with mental disorders is continually growing in contemporary Kyrgyzstan. The data presented by Grzywacz (2010) also testifies to the increase in the popularity of healers in Kazakhstan in the 2000s.

Spiritual healing, biomedicine and the state

As mentioned earlier, the 'discourse of tradition' has been at least partially accepted in the official – governmental and biomedical – attitude to 'folk' medicine. It was expressed in the activities of the Republican Centre of Eastern and Contemporary Medicine in Almaty founded under the auspices of the Ministry of Health. Its main purpose was to institutionalize traditional medicine, to vet traditional practices in order to differentiate 'the wealth of ancient national knowledge' from what was perceived as harmful and connected with the practices of 'charlatans'. This attitude was also characteristic of the physicians working at the Centre whose important obligation was to monitor the healers.

Bureaucratic legitimization procedures initiated by the Centre started with a preliminary assessment of the mental health of the prospective healers carried out by a special commission with the participation of a psychiatrist. According to the Centre's statistics, between 1991 and 1996 as many as 1781 candidates out of 2508 were rejected, 1434 (80.5%) of them because of 'psychiatric disorders' (Khabieva 1997, 9). However, in the opinion of the physicians from the Centre, the 'call of spirits' should be clearly differentiated from mental illness. Not only did they accept it as a part of the Kazakh tradition, but some of them had had the same experiences, as in the case of the deputy director of the Centre, Tamara, a doctor and a healer. As I could observe, various complementary therapies were often practised by medical doctors themselves, and that certainly influenced their approach to traditional healers.[15]

An approved person had to work for two months at the Centre under strict supervision of a doctor and the next stages of her/his career depended on the medical assessment of the results. Candidates were obliged to attend courses at the school for healers opened at the Centre, which provided training in some specialties (folk phytotherapy, bone-setting, bio-energy treatment, parapsychology, astrology and 'cosmic medicine') together with a short course on basic anatomy. The examination commission included, besides some members of the senior staff of the Centre, a representative of the Ministry of Health and a psychiatrist appointed by the Ministry. After passing final examinations, healers got certificates and obtained the right to work legally. However, they were also obliged to pay for a licence and to repeat the procedure every two (later, three) years, a requirement which was not met by many practitioners. Formally, dealing with four types of diseases was forbidden to healers: psychiatric problems; cancer; infectious diseases; and health problems that needed surgical interventions. Besides, healers might be punished[16] for various improprieties, like performing mass séances of treatment or 'using wild methods'. What methods were considered 'wild' depended on the decision of doctors; in the opinion of the head of the division of contemporary medicine it was, for example, beating the patient with a whip, often used in traditional healing.[17] Officials from a special unit at the Centre were given the right to monitor healers from the whole country (although the Centre established its branches in several other *oblast* main cities), yet the controls were not particularly effective and many unlicensed practitioners worked in the cities and even more so in the villages.

The procedure of bureaucratic accreditation was also applied to spiritual healers, who – if successful – got a certificate of *teopsikhoterapevt* ('theopsychotherapist'). All in all, between 1991 and 2000 about 1000 practitioners received certificates of 'a professional folk healer of the Republic of Kazakhstan' in one of four specialties: 'theopsychotherapist'; phytotherapist; bone-setter; and 'bio-energy therapist'. In the case of spiritual healers, obtaining a certificate was, however, often treated as a rather costly formal requirement and sometimes even an obstacle in the way of the healer. Rakhilyam, the shamaness, maintained that it was her great mistake that she had decided to undergo this procedure, because her helping spirits were discontented with that and hindered her further progress. An interplay of different factors could be observed in healers' decision making. On the one hand they wanted to get a more stable position in the market and, in the cities, the opportunity to work in the centres of complementary medicine; yet on the other, both for them and their patients, traditional sources of legitimacy remained the most valued.[18] And the 'call of spirits' was definitely the main constituent of traditional legitimacy, which was also admitted by the physicians from the Centre.

The attitude of those medical specialists who are rather positive about the value of traditional spiritual healing may be illustrated by the statements of a psychiatrist delegated by the Ministry of Health who had worked for several years as a member of the certification commission at the Centre. This Kazakh woman, a professor of psychiatry, expressed her doubts about mental-health assessments and argued for a very careful approach. In her opinion, someone who was diagnosed with schizophrenia might sometimes be 'entirely normal' and apparently deviant behaviour might simply prove the extraordinary abilities of that person, for example, clairvoyant powers. She also maintained that, albeit rare, such special abilities were real, and her experiences at the Centre had significantly changed her viewpoint as a psychiatrist, although it was not shared by the majority of her colleagues from the psychiatric clinic.

According to Kassymbekova:

> Professional medical personnel admit that most patients at psychiatric hospitals only arrived after their psychiatric illnesses had reached an advanced stage. Doctors and nurses may not have much faith in religious psychology, but they often shunt 'no-hope cases' off to healers. They view *taeyip*s as a cultural tradition that people in Shymkent and other communities created, protect, and are comforted by. Some even suggest that *taeyip*s should consider getting formal training, so they can offer more professional help. (2003, 4).

Latypov (2010), in his article about the transformation of mental-health care in Tajikistan, ponders the possibility of accommodation of some local beliefs and practices related to spirits and health, in view of the crisis of Tajik psychiatry. He concludes:

> The healers whom we interviewed in Tajikistan were willing to work in partnership with psychiatrists, but in the words of one of them, 'healers do not have close links with psychiatrists because most doctors do not appreciate alternative[s to bio]medicine yet.' (Latypov 2010, 444).

It is worth stressing that some psychiatrists from neighbouring Kyrgyzstan have already started collaboration with spiritual healers, arguing that traditional healing has unquestionable psychotherapeutic value (Adylov 1999, 2007; Molchanova and Aĭtpaeva 2008; Molchanova et al. 2008). My research in Kazakhstan shows that a similar tendency was present there in the second half of the 1990s, partly motivated by the poor quality and availability of psychiatric care. Data about further developments in this field would be of great value.

Conclusions

In this article I attempted to show that traditional discourse on spiritual healers' initiation – the call of the spirits – has been revived in post-Soviet Kazakhstan. This also applies to many other aspects of traditional healing. As Bellér-Hann rightly argues, 'despite the disruptions and changed circumstances, the claim of modern Central Asian healers to local antecedents (and thereby to tradition) is not unfounded' (2001, 74).

I tried to explain the reasons for the government's acceptance of 'folk' medicine, including spiritual healing, which mainly lies in its interest in the resurgence of Kazakh culture and history, important to the legitimacy of the newly independent state. This context was definitely conducive to the revival of spiritual healing. This phenomenon cannot be treated as 'invented tradition' but rather as 'adapted tradition', in Babadzan's (2000) terms. Similar processes were discussed by Hohmann (2010b) in relation to Uzbekistan, in her study on the strategies of reconstruction of the national identity with the use of traditional medicine based on the heritage of Avicenna. She also points out that this is an instrumental 'rehabilitation' of tradition, rather than invention of tradition. In that case, however, official recognition of traditional medicine is limited only to the so-called 'great tradition' of Avicenna, while in Kazakhstan the reference to 'national heritage' led to the rehabilitation of the entire body of 'folk' medicine.

I focused on 'shamanic illness' and the changing attitude to the 'call of spirits' because it seems exceptional in the sense that it appears the most resilient, the core experience of the spiritual healer which has strikingly uniform traits. I argued that the significance of the remembrance of the dead among the Kazakh and other Turkic peoples contributed to the revival of beliefs about the 'call of spirits'. The strength of this tradition has, in my opinion, helped to restore the previous meaning of the call of spirits in popular discourse and influenced biomedical (mainly psychiatric) discourse, especially, but not exclusively, in the institutional context of the Republican Centre of Eastern and Contemporary Medicine.

The example of 'shamanic illness' is illustrative, because it reveals how political, economic and social transformations influenced the valorization of traditional knowledge, perceptions of illness and healing at the popular and official level. Although in general the position of complementary medicine in Kazakhstan seems stable, the current situation suggests that official policy towards 'folk' medicine may change along with the attempts to develop the state according to modern standards.

Acknowledgements

I would like to thank the anonymous reviewers for insightful comments and constructive suggestions.

Notes

1. I use the term 'spiritual healers' in reference to those practitioners who appeal to spirits (of ancestors and saints) or God in their activities.
2. The first, short version of this paper was presented at the conference 'Healing Paradigms and the Politics of Health in Central Asia' organized by the Global Health Research Center of Central Asia at Columbia University in New York on 8 April 2011.
3. However, there is evidence of the existence of female shamans (see Basilov 1992, 38, 55; Garrone 2000, 138–143; Michaels 2003, 29).
4. Mental illness was commonly ascribed in Central Asia to the influence of evil spirits which were expelled in the course of the shaman's or mullah's healing. See for instance a detailed report by Divaev (1899) of the healing séance of the Kyrgyz (that is, Kazakh) *baqsı* who exorcized *jinns* from the mentally ill patient ('hit by *jinns*').
5. For detailed descriptions of 'shamanic illness' among Turkic and other Central Asian peoples see Dyrenkova (1930) and Basilov (1992, 106–142). It is not, of course, an emic term – the Kazakh usually speak about being pressed or smothered by ancestor spirits. Privratsky quotes the saying: 'The ancestor spirits "burn" in the Kazak healer' (2004, 572).
6. I will not refer further to the well known but discredited and now irrelevant arguments developed long ago by ethnologists and historians of religion about the sources of 'shamanism' in mental illness of the shaman (see Eliade 1951).
7. A good and often cited example is the local treatment of *rishta* (the parasitic worm *Dracunculos medinensis* which causes dracunculosis) confirmed as an effective method by Russian physicians (Kushelevskiĭ 1891, 148–149; Palkin 1967, 478–482; cf. Hohmann 2010a, 328–329). A well-known fact is that Russian medicine adopted Kazakh kumiss (*kımız*) – fermented mare's milk – for treatment of tuberculosis and other lung diseases (Afanas'eva 2008, 130–132; Michaels 2003, 34; Palkin 1967, 528–533).

8. Researchers who write about the introduction of Russian medicine in Central Asia generally agree that it served as an instrument for political legitimization of the Empire (Afanas'eva 2008; Hohmann 2010a; Michaels 2003). However, Afanas'eva (2008, 116) warns against direct application of analytical models like Said's Orientalism to the history of the Russian Empire and criticizes Michaels for overgeneralizations.
9. For example, various forms of acupuncture (called in Russ. *iglorefleksoterapiya*). According to the review of the health system in Kazakhstan (Kulzhanov and Rechel 2007, 108), those methods were formally recognized in the Soviet Union as early as in 1977 and permitted as a part of medical rehabilitation.
10. See Louw (2010) for discussion on the significance of dreams as divine revelations in Kyrgyzstan.
11. There are no apparent differences in the initiation experiences of the healers of different ethnic (Turkic) backgrounds, whereas some elements of healing practices differ; for example, Uighur healers use willow twigs for hitting the patients.
12. This is characteristic of the traditional and also contemporary healer's way that s/he is obliged to concentrate on spiritual development and remove all obstacles in this path. Therefore it is better to divorce if the spouse does not accept this mission than disappoint the spirits.
13. Similarly, healers could be called in their dreams to visit a particular *mazar* in order to get a blessing from the saint connected to that sacred place.
14. Unlike the Uzbeks of Khorezm, where Kehl-Bodrogi did not meet any male *folbin* (healer) (Kehl-Bodrogi 2008, 199).
15. As the doctors from the Centre told me, it was estimated that, all in all, until the year 2000, several thousand physicians in Kazakhstan had completed courses of traditional medicine (Chinese and Korean medicine, hirudotherapy, manual therapies) and perhaps quite a large number of them used those methods in practice. Besides, some doctors combined biomedicine with the methods of 'folk' medicine or healing with bio-energy.
16. Formally, they could be imprisoned for one to three years. In practice, inspectors fined such unlicensed healers and tried to persuade them to pass the procedures of official accreditation.
17. Applying a whip was not forbidden – it could be used for expelling evil spirits, but not for beating the patients. However, many healers working outside the Centre continued traditional methods.
18. Similarly, in Kyrgyzstan and Uzbekistan, as Pelkmans (2005) and Kehl-Bodrogi (2008) showed, spiritual healers were not interested in getting official diplomas and relied entirely on traditional legitimacy.

References

Adylov, D. U. 1999. *Psikhiatricheskie i psikhoterapevticheskie aspekty tselitel'stva v Kyrgyzstane* [Psychiatric and Psychotherapeutic Aspects of Healing in Kyrgyzstan]. Bishkek.

Adylov, D. 2007. "Healing at Mazars: Sources of Healing, Methods of Curative Impact, Types of Healers and Criteria of Their Professional Qualifications." In *Mazar Worship in Kyrgyzstan: Rituals and Practitioners in Talas*, edited by G. Aitpaeva, A. Egemberdieva and M. Toktogulova, 377–394. Bishkek: Aigine Research Center.

Afanas'eva, A. 2008. "'Osvobodit' ot shaĭtanov i sharlatanov': diskursy i praktiki rossiĭskoĭ meditsiny v kazakhskoĭ stepi v XIX veke ['Liberate from Devils and Charlatans': Discourses and Practices of Russian Medicine in the Kazakh Steppe in the XIXth Century]." *Ab Imperio* 4: 113–150.

Alimkhanov, Zh. A. 1978. "Psikhopatologicheskie yavleniya v shamanizme [Psychopatological Phenomena in Shamanism]." In *Ocherki po istorii narodnoĭ mediciny Kazakhstana* [Notes on the History of Folk Medicine of Kazakhstan], edited by T. Sh. Sharmanov and B. A. Atchabarov, 65–76. Alma-Ata: Institut kraevoĭ patologii Minzdrava KazSSR.

Aronson, P. 2007. "Rejecting Professional Medicine in Contemporary Russia." *Vestnik, The Journal of Russian and Asian Studies* 8 May. (Accessed January 15, 2012). http://www.sras.org/rejecting_professional_medicine_in_contemporary_russia.

Babadzan, A. 2000. "Anthropology, Nationalism and 'The Invention of Tradition'." *Anthropological Forum* 10 (2): 131–155.

Basilov, V. N. 1992. *Shamanstvo u narodov Sredneĭ Azii i Kazakhstana* [Shamanism of the Peoples of Central Asia and Kazakhstan]. Moskva: Nauka.

Bellér-Hann, I. 2001. "Rivalry and Solidarity among Uyghur Healers in Kazakhstan." *Inner Asia* 3: 73–98.

Bellér-Hann, I. 2004. "The Micropolitics of a Pilgrimage." In *Central Asia on Display. Proceedings of the 7th Conference of the European Society for Central Asian Studies, 2000 Vienna*, edited by G. Rasuly-Paleczek and J. Katschnig, 325–338. Münster: Lit Verlag.

Brown, J., and N. Rusinova. 2002. "'Curing and Crippling': Biomedical and Alternative Healing in Post-Soviet Russia." *Annals of American Academy of Political and Social Science* 583: 161–170.

DeWeese, D. 1994. *Islamization and Native Religion in the Golden Horde: Baba Tükles and Conversion to Islam in Historical and Epic Tradition*. University Park: Pennsylvania State University Press.

Divaev, A. A. 1899. "Iz oblasti kirgizskikh verovaniĭ. Baksy kak lekar' i koldun (Ėtnografičeskiĭ ocherk) [From the Kyrgyz Beliefs. Baksy as a Doctor and Sorcerer (Ethnographic Notes)]." *Izvestiya Obshchestva Arkheologii, Istorii i Ėtnografii pri Imperatorskom Kazanskom Universitete* 15 (3): 307–341.

Dyrenkova, N. P. 1930. "Poluchenie shamanskogo dara po vozzreniyam turetskikh plemen [Reception of the Shamanic Gift according to the Views of Turkic Tribes]." *Sbornik Muzeya Antropologii i Ėtnografii* 9: 267–291.

Eliade, M. 1951. *Le chamanisme et les techniques archaïques de l'extase*. Paris: Payot.

Garrone, P. 2000. *Chamanisme et islam en Asie Centrale. La baksylyk hier et aujourd'hui* [Shamanism and Islam in Central Asia: Baksylyk Yesterday and Today]. Paris: Libraire d'Amérique et d'Orient, Jean Maisonneuve Successeur.

Goršunova, O. V. 2000. "Tyazhkoe bremya 'shamanskogo dara': sud'ba sovremennoĭ ferganskoĭ *bakhshi* [A Heavy Burden of 'Shamanic Gift': the Fate of a Contemporary *Bakhshi* from Fergana]." In *Shamanskiĭ dar. K 80-letiyu doktora istoricheskikh nauk Anny Vasil'evny Smolyak* [The Shamanic Gift. On the 80th Anniversary of Dr. Anna Vasil'evna Smolyak's Birth], edited by V. I. Kharitonova, 191–204. Moskva: Institut ėtnologii i antropologii im. N.N. Miklukho-Maklaya.

Grzywacz, Z. 2010. "Traditional Kazakh Medicine in Change." *Turkic Studies* [online] 2. (Accessed November 20, 2011). http://www.turkicstudies.amu.edu.pl/turkic_studies_2_2010.pdf.

Hohmann, S. 2007. "Les 'médecins-tabib', une nouvelle catégorie d'acteurs thérapeutiques en Ouzbékistan post-soviétique? [Doctors-Tabib: A New Category of the Therapeutic Actors in Post-Soviet Uzbekistan?]." *Autrepart* 42: 73–90.

Hohmann, S. 2010a. "La médecine moderne au Turkestan russe: un outil au service de la politique colonial [Modern Medicine in Russian Turkestan: a Tool at the Colonial Politics Service]." In *Une colonie pas comme les autres?*, edited by S. Gorshenina and S. Abashin, 319–351. Paris: Editions Complexes.

Hohmann, S. 2010b. "National Identity and Invented Tradition: The Rehabilitation of Traditional Medicine in Post-Soviet Uzbekistan." *The China and Eurasia Quaterly Forum* 8 (3): 129–148.

Humphrey, C. 1999. "Shamans in the City." *Anthropology Today* 15 (3): 3–10.

Jessa, P. 2006a. "Aq Jol Soul Healers: Religious Pluralism and a Contemporary Muslim Movement in Kazakhstan." *Central Asian Survey* 25 (3): 359–371.

Jessa, P. 2006b. "Religious Renewal in Kazakhstan: Redefining 'Unofficial Islam'." In *The Postsocialist Religious Question: Faith and Power in Central Asia and East-Central Europe*, edited by Ch. Hann, and the "Civil Religion" Group, 169–190. Berlin: Lit Verlag.

Kassymbekova, B. 2003. "Turning to the Taeyip." *Transitions Online* 27 Nov. (Accessed November 2, 2011). http://www.tol.org/client/article/11110-turning-to-the-taeyip.html.

Kehl-Bodrogi, K. 2008. "Religion is Not so Strong Here." *Muslim Religious Life in Khorezm after Socialism*. Berlin: Lit Verlag.

Khabieva, T. Kh. 1997. "Rol' Respublikanskogo nauchno-prakticheskogo tsentra vostochnoĭ i sovremennoĭ meditsiny v dal'neĭshem sovershenstvovanii aprobatsii narodnykh tseliteleĭ, ikh teoreticheskoĭ i prakticheskoĭ podgotovke [The Role of the Republican Scientific-Practical Centre of Eastern and Contemporary Medicine in the Advancement of Folk Healers, their Theoretical and Practical Preparation]". In *Traditsionnaya i narodnaya medicina* [Traditional and Folk Medicine] *(materialy I Respublikanskoĭ nauchno-prakticheskoĭ konferentsii*, Almaty, 1–3 oktyabrya 1997 g.*)*. Vol. 1, edited by E. A. Abylkasymov and A. V. Chemeris, 6–10. Almaty: Kazakhskiĭ gosudarstvennyĭ meditsinskiĭ universitet.

Kulzhanov, M., and B. Rechel. 2007. "Kazakhstan: Health System Review." *Health Systems in Transition* 9 (7): 1–158.

Kushelevskiĭ, V. I. 1891. *Materialy dlya medicinskoĭ geografii i sanitarnago opisaniya Ferganskoĭ oblasti* [Materials for Medical Geography and Description of Sanitary Conditions in Fergana Valley]. Vol. 2–3, Novyĭ Margelan.

Latypov, A. 2010. "Healers and Psychiatrists: The Transformation of Mental Health Care in Tajikistan." *Transcultural Psychiatry* 47 (3): 419–451.

Louw, M. E. 2010. "Dreaming up futures: Dream Omens and Magic in Bishkek." *History and Anthropology* 21 (3): 277–292.

Michaels, P. A. 2003. *Curative Powers. Medicine and Empire in Stalin's Central Asia.* Pittsburgh: University of Pittsburgh Press.

Molchanova, E., and G. Aĭtpaeva. 2008. "Ritualy v kyrgyzskoj kul'ture i vozmozhnosti ikh ispol'zovaniya v psikhologicheskoĭ praktike [Rituals in Kyrgyz Culture and the Possibilities of their Implementation in Psychological Practice]." *Academic Review of American University in Central Asia* 5 (1): 75–87.

Molchanova, E. S., Sh. Horne, E. A. Kim, V. I. Ten, N. A. Ashiraliev, G. A. Aitpaeva, and D. E. Pokhilko. 2008. "Status of Counseling and Psychology in Kyrgyzstan." *Academic Review of American University in Central Asia* 5 (1): 57–72. (Accessed November 3 2011). http://elibrary.auca.kg:8080/dspace/bitstream/123456789/234/1/Molchanova%20etc_2008_1.pdf.

Omelicheva, M. Y. 2011. "Islam in Kazakhstan: A Survey of Contemporary Trends and Sources of Securitization." *Central Asian Survey* 30 (2): 243–256.

Palkin, B. N. 1967. *Ocherki istorii mediciny i zdravookhraneniya zapadnoĭ Sibiri i Kazakhstana v period prisoedineniya k Rossii (1716–1868)* [Notes on the History of Medicine and Health Care in Western Siberia and Kazakhstan during the Period of Incorporation to Russia (1716–1868)]. Novosibirsk: Zapadno-Sibirskoe Knizhnoe Izdatel'stvo.

Pelkmans, M. 2005. "Clairvoyants and Healers in Kyrgyzstan. New Guises and Uses of an Old Profession." Paper presented at the workshop organised by Institute of Ethnology and Cultural Anthropology, Adam Mickiewicz University in Poznań and Max Planck Institute for Social Anthropology in Halle: *Popular Religiosity after Socialism,* May 28–30, in Czerniejewo, Poland.

Penkala-Gawecka, D. 2002. "Korean Medicine in Kazakhstan: Ideas, Practices and Patients." *Anthropology and Medicine* 9 (3): 315–336.

Penkala-Gawęcka, D. 2009. "Kazakh Medical Traditions in Present-Day Kazakhstan: Locally Rooted, Regionally and Globally Flavoured." In *Proceedings of the 9th Conference of the European Society for Central Asian Studies, 2005 Cracow,* edited by J. Pstrusińska and T. Gacek, 272–283. Newcastle upon Tyne: Cambridge Scholars.

Privratsky, B. 2001. *Muslim Turkistan: Kazak Religion and Collective Memory.* Richmond: Curzon Press.

Privratsky, B. 2004. "Kazak Shamanism." In *Shamanism: An Encyclopedia of World Beliefs, Practices, and Culture,* edited by M. N. Walter and E. J. Neumann Fridman, 569–573. Santa Barbara, CA: ABC-CLIO.

Rasanayagam, J. 2006. "Healing with Spirits and the Formation of Muslim Selfhood in Post-Soviet Uzbekistan." *Journal of the Royal Anthropological Institute* 12: 377–393.

Roy, O. 2000. *The New Central Asia: The Creation of Nations.* London: I.B. Tauris Publishers.

Sharmanov, T. Sh., and B. A. Atchabarov, eds. 1978. *Ocherki po istorii narodnoĭ mediciny Kazakhstana* [Notes on the History of Folk Medicine of Kazakhstan]. Alma-Ata: Institut kraevoĭ patologii Minzdrava KazSSR.

Toleubaev, A. T. 1997. "Nekotorye obshchie vyvody po shamanstvu kazakhov [Some General Remarks on the Kazakh Shamanism]." In *Istoriya issledovaniĭ kul'tury Kazakhstana* [History of the Studies on the Culture of Kazakhstan], edited by E. Z. Kažibekov, 193–203. Almaty: Qazaq universiteti.

Prohibition, stigma and violence against men who have sex with men: effects on HIV in Central Asia

Alisher Latypov[a,b], Tim Rhodes[c] and Lucy Reynolds[d]

[a]Eurasian Harm Reduction Network, Vilnius, Lithuania; [b]Global Health Research Center of Central Asia (GHRCCA), Columbia University, New York, USA; [c]London School of Hygiene and Tropical Medicine, London, UK; [d]London School of Hygiene and Tropical Medicine, London, UK

Conscious of a paucity of evidence, and drawing upon a combination of historical documentary material, research literature and surveillance data, this paper offers a commentary on the social, historical and HIV contexts affecting men who have sex with men in Central Asia. The authors describe the history of men who have sex with men in the five Central Asian republics, before, during and after the Soviet-imposed legal prohibition, which continues in Turkmenistan and Uzbekistan, the only nations in the World Health Organization Europe region where sex between men remains illegal. This historical context frames contemporary responses to men who have sex with men. Despite long-established homoerotic traditions, modern attitudes to men who have sex with men are marked by great hostility, generating stigmatization of sex between men and discrimination against men suspected of it. The losses following public exposure can be severe: loss of employment; limited/lack of health-care access; and safety from physical and sexual assault. Such hostility creates an environment of increased HIV risk, and constrains the production of reliable HIV evidence. The authors argue that the generation of HIV risk, HIV-prevention responses and HIV evidence are products of their historical and social contexts, and call attention to the urgent need for HIV prevention and structural reforms to protect the health of men who have sex with men in Central Asia.

Introduction

The post-Soviet Central Asian republics have experienced some of the fastest growing HIV epidemics in the world and are now considered a 'hotspot' of the global HIV epidemic (Bobrova et al. 2007; Ferencic et al. 2010; Renton et al. 2006; Thorne et al. 2010). While sharing unsterile drug-injecting equipment remains the key driving force of HIV transmission in the regions of Eastern Europe and Central Asia, men who have sex with men (MSM) are at considerable risk of HIV (Baral et al. 2010). Understanding the context of HIV transmission among MSM in Central Asia, however, is hampered by an extreme paucity of reliable or published evidence on this population, on their health status and risk behaviours (Renton et al. 2006; Wolfe et al. 2008).

The lack of accessible or published epidemiological and behavioural data on MSM and their HIV-related risk behaviour is in large part a product of social conditions. For instance, according to Human Rights Watch (2003, 10), when initial attempts were made to research MSM in Kazakhstan, only two leaders of non-governmental organizations (NGOs) would consent to interviews and MSM, who were asked to participate, declined 'for fear of reprisal or disclosure'. Similarly, studies with a focus on MSM in the regions of Eastern Europe and Central Asia show limited findings from Kazakhstan, Kyrgyzstan and Uzbekistan, and an absence of prevalence or behavioural data from Tajikistan and Turkmenistan (Bozicevic et al. 2009). Recent reviews of HIV in Central Asia (Ferencic et al. 2010; Smolak 2010; Thorne et al. 2010) indicate scant data relating to MSM due to their social marginalization, concluding for instance that they 'constitute one of the most hidden segments of the society' (Ferencic et al. 2010, 22). The most recent relevant study we identified, which focused on non-heterosexual and transgender youth in Kyrgyzstan, confirms a near absence of MSM research within academia (Wilkinson and Kirey 2010).

Given the extreme paucity of research on MSM in Central Asia, we seek to provide a culturally and historically grounded analysis of the roots of the widely reported marginalization of MSM populations in this region. We argue that the domains of prohibition, stigma and violence against MSM are key contextual features of the HIV-risk environment shaping contemporary Central Asia and its responses to HIV prevention and research. We conclude by summarizing data on the epidemiology of HIV among MSM and considering the implications for controlling HIV epidemics linked to MSM. Taken together, our aim is to synthesize available data from a variety of documentary and other sources and to illustrate the ways in which contemporary knowledge of HIV among MSM in Central Asia is inevitably a product of historical and social contexts.

Historical shifts in regulating sexuality in Central Asia

Traditional manifestations of homosexuality in Central Asia

In sharp contrast to the marginalization and stigmatization of homosexuality in contemporary Central Asia, there seems to have been little, if any, shame attached to same-sex relationships in the context of '*bachabozi*' before the establishment of the Soviet Union and the creation of Central Asian republics. Pre-Soviet Central Asia was famous for its dancing boys (*bacha*) and their male lovers (*bachaboz*), who together played the '*bachabozi*' (or '*bachabozlik*' in Uzbek), literally translated as 'boygame'. Baldauf (1990) translates the term as 'boylove', but in a modern Tajik–English dictionary (Jamshedov 2008) it now appears as 'homosexuality' and 'pederasty'. '*Bachabozi*' was an acceptable and popular avenue for sexual and erotic relations and encounters between men, stretching far beyond the settled areas of pre-Soviet Central Asia to other Muslim countries including Iran, Egypt, Pakistan and Turkey (Baldauf 1990; Murray and Roscoe 1997).

A common depiction of dancing boys drawn by the European visitors to Central Asia in the late nineteenth and early twentieth centuries featured young boys at the age of physical puberty (and until the beard was impossible to conceal) displaying their dancing and singing skills. They often had slightly shaven front parts of the head and long flowing locks at the back, sometimes augmented by artificial tresses (Pahlen 1964; Schuyler 1966). Dressed as young girls, in brightly coloured flowing robes, with rings and bracelets on their hands and arms, *bacha*s were much favoured by both the elites and ordinary men throughout different areas of Russian Turkestan, Khiva and Bokhara (Figure 1).

Prohibiting homosexuality in Tsarist and Soviet times

With the conquest of Central Asia by Tsarist Russia in the second half of the nineteenth century, the situation began to change. In numerous books and newspaper articles published by Russian authors over the course of colonial rule, the Russified '*bachebazstvo*' came to be constructed as 'sodomy', 'prostitution' and 'pederasty'; as 'sinful', 'depraved' and 'disgraceful'; and as 'backward' and presented as the result of the Islamic seclusion of indigenous women (Baldauf 1990; fon der Khoven 1900; Kushelevsky 1891; Logofet 1909; Vereschagin 1900).

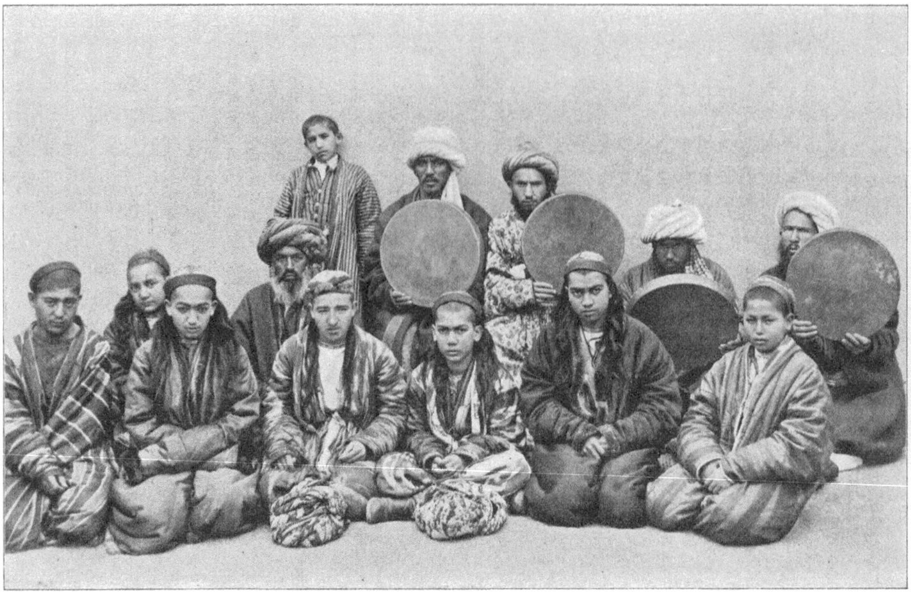

Figure 1. The Royal Troupe of *Bachas* and Musicians in Pre-Soviet Bokhara (Olufsen 1911).

'Playing games with the beardless boys' (*'besaqalbozlik'*) was also lampooned by the first generation of modern Central Asian intellectuals, the *Jadid*s. However, they criticized the practice not because it was forbidden by the Shariat and because the 'morals of individuals were at stake', but because it was a sign of 'degradation' of society and led to 'dereliction of duty to the community' (Khalid 1998, 145–147).

Under the influence of Tsarist administrators, who called for 'rooting out this evil', Muslim clerics had agreed to introduce a ban on the practice. Yet local wealthy Russian settlers had themselves begun to invite dancing boys to perform at their entertainments, and acknowledgements of 'shameful addiction' of some Russians to this 'vice' were not unknown (Kushelevsky 1891; Ostroumov 1896; Sahadeo 2007). Recent historical studies of pre-Soviet Central Asia also proposed that along with bringing in legal female prostitution and the sale of alcohol, Russian rule had made the *bachebazstvo* even more widespread (Khalid 1998).

While the demonization of dancing boys had been part of the Russian 'civilizing-mission' agenda in pre-revolutionary Central Asia, the Bolsheviks lifted this to a new level by launching both penal measures and propaganda campaigns against it. As Soviet Central Asian republics adopted their first criminal codes broadly modelled after the 1922 Russian Criminal Code, *bachabozlik* was criminalized and interpreted exclusively in the context of 'sodomy'. Such interpretation had stripped the *bachabozlik* of its cultural meanings and erotic manifestations that did not involve male sexual relations. The Bolsheviks' categorization of the Central Asian *bachebazstvo* crime as a 'survival of primitive everyday life' in Central Asia also signalled a significant departure from the 'language of modernity' used in European territories of the Soviet Union, where male sexuality was described in terms related to the remits of public health and order (Healey 2001). It placed an emphasis on the social construction of male same-sex love while inverting the gendering of the Russian legislation and prohibiting sexual harassment of young males, who were viewed as victims.

To eliminate this 'vestige of the backward past' and cut its 'social' roots, the Uzbek SSR Criminal Code, which was first adopted in 1926 and was also applicable in Tajikistan until

June 1935, contained the most detailed proscriptions against male same-sex relations (Healey 2001; Karev 1957). Article 280 defined '*bachebazstvo*' as 'the maintenance of persons of the male sex (*bachas*) for *muzhelozhstvo* [sodomy]' and made it punishable with up to five years of imprisonment when the *bacha* was an adult man, and eight years when he was a minor. Other practices prohibited by the Uzbek Criminal Code included the 'preparation and education of *bachas* for sodomy', 'the organization of public entertainments (*bazmy*) with the participation of *bachas*', 'procurement and recruitment of men for sodomy' and 'agreements and contracts between those who maintained *bachas* and the parents or guardians who sold their sons into *bachebazstvo*'. The Turkmen SSR Criminal Code, first adopted in 1927, contained less detailed provisions (Healey 2001; Karev 1957).

In the local Uzbek press of the early 1920s, *bachabozlik* was primarily exposed in humoristic-satirical tones, with one cartoon placing it, along with gambling and womanizing, in the context of depravity (Baldauf 1988). In the late 1920s, as Baldauf (1990) noted, the overarching concern with the *bachaboz* as a symbol of 'everlasting backwardness' was complemented by a modernized package of stereotypes, which demonized the *bachaboz* with the purpose of promoting various political agendas. In 1925, the *bachaboz* 'undermines Lenin's New Economic Policy'; in 1927, he is 'the *mullo–eshon*, the personal union of religious and spiritual-mystical leader, who thwarts the modern school-system and – in addition to boys – thinks of nothing but women (!) and drinking"; in 1928 the *bachaboz* is a 'bureaucrat', who 'is just in time to block the new measures at the beginning of collectivization'; finally, he is featured as a 'modern', 'social parasite who abuses all the offices that are entrusted to him, and on top of that is also a *bachaboz*' (Baldauf 1990, 28–29). However, against the backdrop of the politics of anti-*bachabozlik* propaganda, Soviet ethnographers could still observe the performances of dancing boys at festivities of Tajiks and Uzbeks in the late 1920s (Peschereva 1927).

The Soviet prohibition of male same-sex relations in Central Asia was complete by 1934, after all union republics amended their criminal codes, criminalizing sex between *consenting* adult men and making consensual sodomy illegal. However, mentioning the subject of the Central Asian '*bachebazstvo*' became a taboo even before the introduction of these changes in law, and was last openly discussed by the chairman of the Central Committee of the Uzbek Communist Party in 1932 (Baldauf 1990).

The decriminalization of consensual male same-sex relations in Russia took place in 1993, nearly 60 years after the adoption of the 1934 anti-sodomy legislation, and was followed by decriminalization in 1997 in Kazakhstan and in 1998 in the Kyrgyz Republic and Tajikistan. Sex between consenting males remains illegal however in both Turkmenistan and Uzbekistan (ILGA 2010). In fact, the present-day Uzbek Criminal code continues to employ the pre-Soviet and early Soviet formulations such as 'playing games with the beardless boys', though now defining *besoqolbozlik* as 'voluntary sexual intercourse of two male individuals' to be punished with up to three years of imprisonment (ILGA 2010, 30; Karev 1957).

The social and sexual hierarchy of Soviet prisons

Although the culture of the Gulag was fundamental to the perception of male same-sex relations in prisons and in Soviet society, this culture itself had some of its roots in pre-1930s prison culture. Existing evidence suggests that men who were available for receptive anal sex were treated with brutality already in pre-revolutionary, Tsarist prisons. With the creation and expansion of the Gulag system, the worst features of the sexual subculture of male prisons were retained and reinforced (Healey 2001).

As the system of hierarchy among criminals developed, 'passive' sexually accessible men were incorporated into the lowest social status group of 'pederasts' who were regarded as 'untouchables'. In the 1930s, according to Kuznetsov (1979), in some large prisons 'passive pederasts' had to live in separate barracks which often served as brothels. It was not only those who were convicted of sodomy or seduced by fellow prisoners who were regarded as 'pederasts'. Inmates who violated the prisoners' code of norms were also 'lowered' to this degraded status. The most common routes to the 'pederast' caste included losing at cards and failing to settle debts within the set time, informing on other prisoners to the prison administration, and stealing from fellow inmates (Healey 2001; Kozlovsky 1986; Baldaev, Vasiliev, and Plutser–Sarno 2003, 2006; Baldaev, Vasiliev, and Sidorov 2008). Some authors suggest that in the 1930s and 1940s, prison authorities were encouraging criminals to forcibly sodomize political prisoners, with initiatory rape serving as a means to relegate a man to the caste of 'pederasts' (Baldaev, Vasiliev, and Plutser–Sarno 2006). In the late 1950s and 1960s, prisoners who were not 'legitimate thieves' (*'vor v zakone'*) but dared to present themselves as 'legitimates' or to make other undeserved claims in regard to their status in the criminal hierarchy were often relegated to the untouchable caste (Sidorov 2008). According to Sidorov (2008), by the late 1960s, the number of inmates 'lowered' and 'shamed' for illegitimately claiming an undeserved status was so great that they began to revolt against the 'legitimate thieves', which at some point even led to the establishment of a rule of 'no punishment with the penis' as far as this particular group was concerned (41).

The most common way to relegate a man to the status of 'pederast' was to rape him, but the use of specifically feminizing insults and forcing a man to touch a fellow prisoner's penis with his lips were also sufficient to consign violators of the prisoners' moral code to this caste (Healey 2001; Kozlovsky 1986). Once his new status was established, a man would become 'untouchable' with the exception of those occasions when he was subjected to oral and anal penetration. These physically and morally abused and humiliated people were 'rejected and kicked by other prisoners' (Baldaev, Vasiliev, and Sidorov 2008, 254). They were forced to eat from their own 'crockery and spoons, marked with drilled holes' and washed separately from other dishes (Baldaev, Vasiliev, and Plutser–Sarno 2003, 214). The prison code of morals forbade touching these people or taking anything from them (Kuznetsov 1979). They had to 'sit at designated seats in the canteen, and stand in designated places during morning and evening calls'; they did 'the dirtiest, lowest jobs in the prison' and were 'slaves of the slaves' (Baldaev, Vasiliev, and Sidorov 2008, 254).

Men imprisoned through the anti-sodomy legislation as well as those who were otherwise relegated to untouchable status by fellow inmates were marked with special tattoos, often applied forcibly to the back, buttocks, forehead, cheeks, ears or the upper lip (Baldaev, Vasiliev, and Plutser–Sarno 2003, 2006; Baldaev, Vasiliev, and Sidorov 2008; Bronnikov and Bronnikov 2003).

Stigma and violence against men who have sex with men in modern Central Asia

In this section, we look at stigma and violence against MSM in contemporary Central Asia in both community and prison settings to precede the review of the HIV epidemiological situation amongst MSM and to support our concluding discussion on the generation of HIV knowledge and implications for controlling the epidemic.

In everyday life

A substantial part of the information that was collected on discrimination and violence against MSM in post-Soviet Central Asian republics concerns Kyrgyzstan. This, to some extent, can be explained by the fact that this country has had the strongest group of NGO activists devoted to the rights and needs of lesbian, gay, bisexual and transgender persons, as well as an enabling socio-political context including donor activity.

Evidence that has emerged from Kyrgyzstan in the past decade suggests that the local society's perception of homosexuality is highly negative and hostile, very often manifesting itself in discrimination, hatred and physical and psychological violence against MSM. Men can be fired from their jobs or refused work because of their sexual orientation as well as turned away by the staff of cafés, restaurants, clubs, shops and other service providers. Offensive and disparaging remarks from the public are considered 'normal things' and few MSM are able and willing to speak about their sexual identity publicly (van der Veur 2004).

The 'everyday humiliations' of non-heterosexual people in Kyrgyzstan and Tajikistan extend to violence from family members, with MSM being often forcefully married to women or planning to get married because of family pressures (HRW 2008; Universal Periodic Review Submission on Sexual Rights in Tajikistan 2011). One study notes a man who reported that because he was 'homosexual his family stoned him and his brother cut his neck with a knife' (OSI 2007, 15). In this context, coming out to families is often impossible. In the words of one man from Southern Kyrgyzstan recorded by the same study:

> I am already 30 and still have not told anybody about [my] sexual orientation. If I try to tell my parents then I simply would not have any other choice but to hang myself. (OSI 2007, 13)

The same study found that 78% of a sample of 49 MSM reported experiencing persecution, with the remaining 22% declining to respond. Of those who were persecuted in one way or another, 14% reported being the victims of rape. When any forms of persecution took place, the majority of men (88%) did not complain to the authorities (OSI, 2007).

Furthermore, there are multiple reports on the abuse and harassment of populations at risk of HIV infection, such as sex workers and drug users, by the police in post-Soviet Central Asian republics (Ibragimov et al. 2011; HRW 2003; Latypov 2008). In Tajikistan, research on this topic to date is limited, with one recent study noting the police specifically targeting MSM meeting places in order to harass and extort money from them (Vinogradov 2008). There are also published reports of Tajik police targeting MSM and blackmailing them into identifying other MSM (UNOCHA IRIN 2004).

In Kyrgyzstan also, a police presence at MSM meeting places has been noted as offering opportunities to 'harass and extort money from those who gather there' (OSI 2007, 17). Based on reports on MSM in Kyrgyzstan, we can identify a variety of policing practices that appear fundamental to the oppressed status of MSM, their distrust and fear of the police. First, extortion and blackmail are reportedly commonplace. Often richer men are targeted as victims, but other MSM also report having to pay police bribes. On some occasions, when, following their unjustified detention, young MSM are unable to pay the police, they are forced to 'sexually entertain police officers' (van der Veur 2004, 29).

Second, unjustified arrests and detentions of MSM are reported (HRW 2008; OSI 2007; van der Veur 2004). As one man from Kyrgyzstan stated:

> [The p]olice persecute me and they have arrested me several times. I have been beaten and threatened many times while I was staying in the police department for the sole reason that I am gay. (van der Veur 2004, 5)

Third, when police officers arrest MSM, this can be followed by physical violence, rape or abuse, as the accounts extracted from one study illustrate:

> I came back from a disco and stopped the taxi. When we left, a little car overtook us and crossed the road. The machine was left by two policemen and they ordered me to sit in their car . . . They began to interrogate me – am I gay or not, what was I doing in the gay club. Then they began to beat me and to demand to tell the names and phones of my familiars who are gays. I suffered all this. Then they forced me to give oral sex. (van der Veur 2004, 27–28)

In prisons

In the Kyrgyz Republic, a study was conducted among 112 inmates who were excluded by the prison sub-culture in six correctional colonies in 2009. According to this study, between 2% and 4.5% of prisoners in this country may belong to the stigmatized and discriminated group of 'relegated' or 'outcast' ('*obizhennye*') MSM (Harm Reduction Association 2009). As in Soviet times, the main routes to the 'outcast' caste include initiatory rape, losing at cards and failing to pay the debt, theft, informing or complaining about other inmates to the prison administration. This caste is segregated from other inmates socially, though accessible sexually. They are normally dressed in rags and have to do all the 'dirty' work in barracks such as cleaning the toilets. It is forbidden for these men to communicate and to eat meals together with other inmates, to go to common bathrooms, to visit meeting rooms or to pray in common prayer rooms with other inmates (Harm Reduction Association 2009). The same study suggests that '*avtoritety*' (prison-gang leaders) introduced the rule that 'decent' men should not use narcotic drugs in prisons. In effect, this rule implied that inmates who continued using drugs or who might initiate drug use were mainly those people who were relegated to the status of '*obizhennye*'. Although harm-reduction services were available in colonies, men excluded by the prison subculture were reluctant to get sterile injecting equipment from these services due to the fear of punishment (Harm Reduction Association 2009).

In Tajikistan, according to the assessment of harm-reduction needs conducted in five correctional facilities in 2006, male same-sex relations are strongly discouraged by religious *avtoritety*, who promote spiritual cleanliness and the practice of self-improvement and tolerate neither drug use nor sex between males. Men who practise 'passive' receptive sex with other men are considered the lowest caste. They are abused, stigmatized and discriminated against as in Kyrgyzstan. Male same-sex relations in prisons are also forbidden by the Tajik prison administration. These formal and informal prohibitions and stigmas can largely explain why between 10% and 20% of adults and as many as half of male juvenile offenders, who were estimated to have sex with other male inmates, often avoid possessing a condom and asking for condoms from harm-reduction service providers at the so-called 'friendly rooms' (Khidirov et al. 2006). According to Khidirov and others (2006), many inmates 'are aware of the routes of transmission of HIV and sexually transmitted infections (STIs), know that because of their risk behaviour they are vulnerable to STIs and HIV infection, but all the same, do not use condoms with same-sex partners' (12). At the same time, only 10% of inmates were estimated to use condoms with their female partners during conjugal visits to prisons. As study participants explained, a man insisting on using a condom puts himself at risk of being suspected by his wife to have had an unprotected sex with other men, to have 'practiced homosexuality', and to have contracted an STI. A wife asking her husband to use a condom is equally at risk of being accused of committing adultery (Khidirov et al. 2006).

HIV epidemic situation and risk behaviours amongst MSM

Kazakhstan

As of the end of August 2010, Kazakh authorities reported a total of 15,151 cumulative cases of diagnosed HIV infection. Seventy-five of these cases (0.5%) were diagnosed in MSM (Kul'zhanova 2010). On the basis of findings from rapid assessment studies, the government estimates that there are 37,500 MSM in the country (Ismailova 2010).

In the 2010 integrated bio-behavioural study among MSM, the prevalence of HIV in the total sample was 1%, whereas among MSM who reported injecting drug use the prevalence of HIV was 10% (Tukeyev et al. 2011). According to the 2009 integrated bio-behavioural study among 880 MSM, the prevalence of HIV was 0.3%, 3.9% of the sample had hepatitis C virus (HCV), and 5.2% were infected with syphilis (Government of Kazakhstan 2010; Tukeyev 2010). Self-reported history of accessing any HIV-prevention programmes at least once in the past six months was high, reaching 68% in 2009. Population Services International (PSI) (2010) carried out a respondent-driven sample study of 289 MSM residents in Almaty in 2010. Respondents reported a mean of 10.3 sexual partners in the past year; of these, 9.4, on average, were male. Unsafe vaginal or anal sex was reported with regular partners by 79.2%, with casual partners by 44.9%, and with commercial partners by 18.4%.

The Global Fund to Fight AIDS, Tuberculosis and Malaria (the Global Fund) provides the bulk of the funding for prevention activities for MSM in Kazakhstan. Twenty-nine MSM-friendly free-of-charge confidential clinics providing services primarily to people who inject drugs and sex workers have been set up in some regions of the country. In 2009, 22,021 clients visited these clinics including 415 MSM, representing less than 2% of the clientele (Government of Kazakhstan 2010) and reflecting, perhaps, both underreporting of MSM status and the reluctance/inability of MSM to use those services. According to a focus group discussion conducted recently in Almaty with 11 MSM, most of these men contacted private clinics or paid for medical services. They also suggested that their full-time jobs prevented them from accessing free 'friendly cabinets' which had limited hours of operations and were closed on weekends (Deryabina, Osipov, and Surdina 2011).

Kyrgyzstan

In 2005, Oostvogels suggested that the estimated number of MSM in Kyrgyzstan might range from 18,000 to 36,000, or 1–2% of the sexually active male population (Oostvogels 2005). This estimate was later accepted and reported by the Government of Kyrgyzstan (2006).

The first HIV case in a man who had sex with men was diagnosed by the Kyrgyz authorities in 2007 (Government of Kyrgyzstan 2008). According to a recent study conducted by the AIDS Centre in 2008 among 84 MSM, the prevalence of HIV infection in this sample was 1.2%; moreover, 1.2% were also infected with HCV, and 10.7% had syphilis. Eighty-two per cent of respondents reported having two or more sexual partners in the three months before the interview. Forty-nine per cent were reached with HIV-prevention activities (often condoms or information and education materials) at least once in the past six months, and about half (52%) had an HIV test in the past year (Ismailova 2010).

In an earlier study involving 49 MSM and conducted in 2006 in the cities of Bishkek, Osh and Jalal-Abad, 80% reported having anal sexual intercourse in the past six months. Among them, only 20% always used condoms; thirty-five per cent used condoms from time to time; ten per cent used condoms only with occasional partners and 27.5% responded that they usually did not use condoms during anal intercourse (OSI 2007).

HIV-prevention services available in Kyrgyzstan by 2010 included the promotion of safer sex and HIV testing, condom distribution, a hotline, and the provision of a shelter for needy MSM. There were two MSM-friendly clinics in Bishkek. Rough estimates suggested that several hundred MSM, across Bishkek, Osh and Karabalta, might have been in receipt of safer sex, HIV-testing and condom-distribution services.

Tajikistan

Until 2011, no integrated bio-behavioural study among MSM has been conducted in Tajikistan. Although none of the cumulative 2336 cases of HIV infection diagnosed in the country by October 2010 was reported as homosexually transmitted, the government believes that this was due to the lack of access to the hard-to-reach population of MSM (Republican AIDS

Centre 2010; Government of Tajikistan 2010). In a cross-sectional study conducted among 491 active injecting drug users in Dushanbe in 2004, none of the 21 men reporting a lifetime history of sex with men was HIV positive (Beyrer et al. 2009). No scientifically robust studies to estimate the size of the MSM population have been conducted before 2011, and the only available estimate of 58,000 MSM in Tajikistan was proposed on the basis of author's assumption that at minimum 4% of sexually active men are MSM (Vinogradov 2008).

Against the backdrop of the lack of HIV-prevalence data, several recent studies shed more light on the HIV-risk behaviours of MSM in Tajikistan. In a 2004 study conducted among 145 MSM in Dushanbe, 87% of respondents recruited through convenience sampling reported a lifetime history of having unprotected sex with men; fifty per cent suggested that they had never or very rarely used condoms; and more than one third of participants (n = 56) reported having traded sex for money (Gulov and Pirov 2004). In another multi-site study conducted in five cities and four districts (n = 200), 13.5% reported a lifetime history of drug use, 14.5% never used condoms with men in the past year and 25.5% reported occasional condom use with men in the past 12 months. A large proportion of men in this study (73%) reported having sex with women (Vinogradov 2008). The 2010 PSI respondent-driven sample study incorporated 289 MSM living in Dushanbe. In this sample, there were 43 respondents who had more than 100 male sexual partners and 16 respondents who had more than 30 female sexual partners in the past 12 months.

The Global Fund and PSI have funded two NGOs for outreach, which provide referrals to STI treatment, voluntary counselling and testing services, and distribute educational materials, condoms and lubricants in Dushanbe.

Turkmenistan

In Turkmenistan, research and surveillance data on MSM to date is extremely limited.

The Government of Turkmenistan denies the existence of the HIV/AIDS problem in the country, reporting a cumulative total of only two cases to the WHO and UNAIDS (MSF 2010). According to MSF (2010), despite the change in the leadership of the country, local government officials continue to reassure external visitors that there are no cases of HIV in Turkmenistan and to claim that 'if there were HIV-positive individuals in Turkmenistan, then they would, of course, receive treatment according to international standards' (11). However, unofficial sources suggest that there might be a substantial and unaddressed epidemic in the country (MSF 2010).

There are six HIV-prevention centres in Turkmenistan. They test blood donors and those with symptoms which could be HIV-related, but no specific prevention initiatives have been targeted at MSM in the National AIDS Plan.

Uzbekistan

While data on MSM in Uzbekistan is limited, information formally released by the Uzbek government suggests that integrated bio-behavioural studies among MSM have been conducted regularly since 2005, albeit in the capital city of Tashkent alone. The first study in 2005 (n = 102, convenience sample) suggested a well-established HIV epidemic among MSM, in turn raising questions about potential levels of HIV prevalence elsewhere in the country: HIV prevalence was 10.8%, HCV 11% and syphilis 8%. In this study, the rate of condom use with the regular partner at last sexual intercourse was 39%; thirty-eight per cent reported female partners, with whom 58% had used condoms. Only 26% reported having been HIV tested in the past 12 months (Uzbekistan Multisectoral Expert Council 2010).

However, a more recent integrated bio-behavioural study among MSM in Tashkent, conducted in 2009, found an HIV prevalence of 6.8% (Government of Uzbekistan 2010). According to this study, 44.1% of respondents had been HIV tested in the past year, 41.5% were reached with HIV prevention activities, and 87.3% reported condom use during the last anal intercourse (Government of Uzbekistan 2010). Although no data were available for other cities, one cross-sectional study conducted in Samarkand in 2004–5 involving 43 male sex workers recorded that 7% had a self-reported lifetime history of injecting drugs, 2.3% shared drugs with their clients, and only 2.3% always used condoms with their clients (Todd et al. 2009).

The coverage of HIV prevention among MSM appears very limited and largely confined to the capital city of Tashkent. Two NGOs (ANTIAIDS and Munavar Tong) were active as of 2010, funded by the Global Fund. They were able to provide limited counselling, outreach, distribution of educational materials and condoms.

Implications for HIV epidemic control

By combining a narrative review of documentary and research evidence we have sought to illuminate how historical shifts in Central Asia have regulated MSM, which, in turn, may shape how social contexts of structural and everyday violence affecting MSM contemporaneously impact upon HIV risk as well as the generation of HIV evidence. We do not purport to identify how past processes in the regulation of sexuality affect current HIV responses, because the paucity of data precludes this type of analysis. Rather, our aim has been to review the data that are available on the history of MSM and HIV in the region, and in doing so, contextualize an interpretation of what little is currently known about the epidemiology of HIV among MSM.

The combination of evidence we reviewed suggests that HIV is present, and in some Central Asian settings well established in MSM networks, and that reported levels of risk behaviour are sufficient to maintain transmission. While HIV epidemics in the region remain driven by injecting drug use (Thorne et al. 2010), we draw attention to the danger that growing concentrated epidemics among MSM remain concealed by the paucity of evidence available. Our review suggests that the paucity and uncertain reliability of epidemiological evidence pertaining to MSM is a reflection of broader social conditions and the structural inequalities these reproduce. Social stigma linked to men having sex with men appears pervasive since the time of early Soviet Central Asia, despite an alternative historical reading prior to the Bolshevik's 'modernization' project to 'root out the remnants of the backward past'. This manifests itself throughout various layers of society – from national responses to family relations – but is arguably most apparent when it combines with the force of the law and everyday policing practices. With the losses and harms of disclosure both severe and likely, there appears a strong (justifiable) tendency of avoidance or denial when attempts are made to survey or research MSM risk behaviour (HRW 2003; OSI 2007). Moreover, attempts may be made at the level of the nation-state to deny the existence of MSM and HIV, as appears to be the case currently in Turkmenistan (MSF 2010). The social conditions regulating MSM practices shape what is known about HIV as well as what is knowable.

Furthermore, despite the major constraints these social conditions place upon documenting how MSM and HIV risk is experienced from the perspectives of those affected, our review provides sufficient evidence to indicate how HIV risk is increased as a result of structural violence (Farmer et al. 1996). For instance, public prejudice limits access to HIV testing, counselling and prevention information, since most MSM fear identification if they are seen in a public place perceived as associated with gay men. The potential consequences of HIV exposure range from social rejection to fatal assault. With reports of police harassment, physical abuse, extortion and blackmail being very common, the policing practices effectively exacerbate the situation rather than providing protection from violence against MSM. Similar observations have been made elsewhere, including how the policing of HIV-affected populations reflects broader and deep-seated neuroses or risk concerns in a society (Rhodes et al. 2008; Sarang et al. 2010).

Most directly, the illegality of sex between consenting men in Turkmenistan and Uzbekistan serves as a fundamental obstacle to enabling the conditions where MSM have the means and capacity to enact their HIV-risk avoidance. Instead, the emphasis on the criminalization of sex between men feeds an HIV-risk environment in prisons and detention centres in which MSM often become subjected to forced unprotected receptive intercourse with multiple people, with obvious dangers for onwards HIV transmission. Reported risk practices from Kyrgyz and Tajik penitentiary facilities are alarming. The available data we reviewed indicate an urgent need to research and develop HIV-prevention interventions in Central Asian prison settings. Evidence internationally substantiates how detention facilities act as a major structural factor in the distribution of HIV and in the undermining of individual agency towards HIV prevention (Beyrer et al. 2003; Open Society Foundations 2011).

Finally, without long-term well-designed anti-stigma and discrimination campaigns targeting various audiences, as well as parallel national and regional advocacy activities aimed at legal reform and policy change, there is a serious likelihood that many of the on-going prevention interventions will have only a very limited impact. The governments of Central Asian republics must therefore urgently recognize the vulnerability of MSM to the HIV epidemic and the significance of historically, culturally and socially constructed HIV risk environment in the region. This recognition should materialize in both financial and political commitments to expand the evidence base, mitigate individual and structural risk factors and implement interventions that are grounded in local contextual realities of these republics.

Acknowledgements

The authors would like to acknowledge the contributions made to this work by Catherine Dodds at Sigma Research, London School of Hygiene and Tropical Medicine, Elizabeth Costenbader at FHI 360, William Zule at RTI International, and Roman Dudnik at AIDS Foundation East–West.

References

Baldaev, D., S. Vasiliev, and A. Plutser–Sarno. 2003. *Russian Criminal Tattoo Encyclopaedia*, Vol. I. Göttingen: Fuel.

Baldaev, D., S. Vasiliev, and A. Plutser–Sarno. 2006. *Russian Criminal Tattoo Encyclopaedia*, Vol. II. Göttingen: Fuel.

Baldaev, D., S. Vasiliev, and A. Sidorov. 2008. *Russian Criminal Tattoo Encyclopaedia*, Vol. III. Göttingen: Fuel.

Baldauf, I. 1988. "Die Knabenliebe in Mittelasien: Bacabozlik." *Ethnizität und Gesellschaft Occasional Papers* 17.

Baldauf, I. 1990. "*Bacabozlik*: Boylove, Folksong and Literature in Central Asia." *Paidika* 2 (2): 12–31.

Baral, S., D. Kizub, N. Masenior, A. Peryskina, J. Stachowiak, M. Stibich, V. Moguilny, and C. Beyrer. 2010. "Male Sex Workers in Moscow, Russia: A Pilot Study of Demographics, Substance Use Patterns, and Prevalence of HIV-1 and Sexually Transmitted Infections." *AIDS Care* 22 (1): 112–118.

Beyrer, C., J. Juttiwutikarn, W. Teokul, M. Razak, V. Suriyanon, N. Srirak, T. Vongchuk, S. Tovanabutra, T. Sripaipan, and D. Celentano. 2003. "Drug Use, Increasing Incarceration Rates, and Prison Associated HIV risks in Thailand." *AIDS and Behavior* 7 (2): 153–161.

Beyrer, C., Z. Patel, J. Stachowiak, F. Tishkova, M. Stibich, L. Eyzaguirre, and J. Carr, et al. 2009. "Characterization of the Emerging HIV Type 1 and HCV Epidemics Among Injecting Drug Users in Dushanbe, Tajikistan." *AIDS Research and Human Retroviruses* 25 (9): 853–860.

Bobrova, N., A. Sarang, R. Stuikyte, and K. Lezhentsev. 2007. "Obstacles in Provision of Anti-Retroviral Treatment to Drug Users in Central and Eastern Europe and Central Asia: A Regional Overview." *The International Journal of Drug Policy* 18 (4): 313–318.

Bozicevic, I., L. Voncina, L. Zigrovic, M. Munz, and J. Lazarus. 2009. "HIV Epidemics Among Men Who Have Sex With Men in Central and Eastern Europe." *Sexually Transmitted Infections* 85 (5): 336–342.

Bronnikov, A., and D. Bronnikov. 2003. *Tatuirovka za Reshetkoi*. Perm': Prikamskii Sotsial'nyi Institut.

Deryabina, A., K. Osipov, and T. Surdina. 2011. *Mapping of Key HIV/AIDS Services, Assessment of Their Quality, and Analysis of Gaps and Needs of Most-at-Risk Populations in Selected Sites of Kazakhstan*. Arlington, VA: United States Agency for International Development.

Farmer, P., M. Connors, and J. Simmons. 1996. *Women, Poverty and AIDS*. Monroe, ME: Common Courage Press.

Ferencic, N., R. Malyuta, P. Nary, J. Mimica, A. Adams, and A. Winter. 2010. *Blame and Banishment: The Underground HIV Epidemic Affecting Children in Eastern Europe and Central Asia*. Geneva: The United Nations Children's Fund.

fon der Khoven, N. 1900. "O Polovykh Izvrascheniiakh na Vostoke." *Obozrenie Psikhiatrii, Nevrologii, i Eksperimental'noi Psikhologii* 6: 422–426.

Government of Kazakhstan. 2010. "UNGASS Country Progress Report." Reporting Period: January 2008–December 2009. Almaty.

Government of Kyrgyzstan. 2006. "State Programme on Prevention of HIV/AIDS Epidemic and Its Socio-Economic Consequences in Kyrgyz Republic for The Years 2006–2010." Bishkek.

Government of Kyrgyzstan. 2008. "UNGASS Country Progress Report." Reporting Period: January 2006–December 2007. Bishkek.

Government of Kyrgyzstan. 2010. "UNGASS Country Progress Report." Reporting Period: January 2008–December 2009. Bishkek.

Government of Tajikistan. 2010. "UNGASS Country Progress Report." Reporting Period: January 2008–December 2009. Dushanbe.

Government of Uzbekistan. 2010. "UNGASS Country Progress Report." Reporting Period: January 2008–December 2009. Tashkent.

Gulov, K., and D. Pirov. 2004. *Analytical Report on Advocacy and Prevention of HIV/AIDS Among Men Who Have Sex With Men*. Dushanbe: Centre for Legal Support of Youth.

Harm Reduction Association. 2009. *Rapid Assessment of Behavioral Aspects of HIV/AIDS/STIs and Accessibility of Harm Reduction Services Among People "Outcasted by The Prison Sub-Culture" in Colonies 3, 31, 8, 16, 1, 27–For Subsequent Provision of Specialized HIV Prevention Services to This Category of Convicted People*. Bishkek: Harm Reduction Association.

Healey, D. 2001. *Homosexual Desire in Revolutionary Russia: The Regulation of Sexual and Gender Dissent*. Chicago: The University of Chicago Press.

HRW. 2003. *Fanning The Flames: How Human Rights Abuses Are Fueling The AIDS Epidemic in Kazakhstan*. New York: Human Rights Watch 15, no. 4 (D).

HRW. 2008. *These Everyday Humiliations: Violence Against Lesbians, Bisexual Women, and Transgender Men in Kyrgyzstan*. New York: Human Rights Watch.

Ibragimov, U., E. Khasanova, A. Latypov, and P. Dzhamolov. 2011. *The Needs of Opiate Users in Dushanbe in 2010: A Qualitative Assessment*. Dushanbe: SPIN Plus.

ILGA. 2010. *State-Sponsored Homophobia: A World Survey of Laws Prohibiting Same Sex Activity Between Consenting Adults*. Brussels: The International Lesbian, Gay, Bisexual, Trans and Intersex Association.

Ismailova, A. 2010. "The Analysis of The Situation Related to HIV Infection Among MSM in Central Asia, 2010." Presented at the regional conference on "The HIV epidemic in Central Asia: Further development of epidemiological surveillance," 18–19 May, in Almaty, Kazakhstan.

Jamshedov, P. 2008. *Tajik-English Dictionary*. Dushanbe: Academy of Sciences of the Republic of Tajikistan.

Karev, D., ed. 1957. *Ugolovnoe Zakonodatel'stvo SSSR i Soiuznykh Respublik. Sbornik (Osnovnye Zakonodatel'nye Akty)*. Moscow: Gosudarstvennoe Izdatel'stvo Iuridicheskoi Literatury.

Khalid, A. 1998. *The Politics of Muslim Cultural Reform: Jadidism in Central Asia*. Berkeley: University of California Press.

Khidirov, M., R. Nurov, M. Rakhmanova, A. Mirzoev, and V. Magkoev. 2006. "Report on The Results of Assessment of Introduction of Harm Reduction Programmes in The Correctional Institutions of the

Department of Correctional Affairs of the Ministry of Justice of the Republic of Tajikistan". Dushanbe.
Kozlovksy, V. 1986. *Argo Russkoi Gomoseksual'noi Subkul'tury: Materialy k Izucheniiu*. Benson, VT: Chalidze Publications.
Kul'zhanova, D. 2010. HIV/AIDS Epidemiological Situation in August 2010, During Eight Months of 2010, and by September 1, 2010. Unpublished document.
Kushelevsky, V. 1891. *Materialy Dlia Meditsinskoi Geografii i Sanitarnogo Opisaniia Ferganskoi Oblasti*, Vol. II. Novyi Margelan: Izdanie Ferganskogo Oblastnogo Statisticheskago Komiteta.
Kuznetsov, E. 1979. *Mordovsky Marathon*. Jerusalem. Reprinted in Kozlovksy, V. 1986. *Argo Russkoi Gomoseksual'noi Subkul'tury: Materialy k Izucheniiu*, 200–210. Benson, VT: Chalidze Publications.
Latypov, A. 2008. "Two Decades of HIV/AIDS in Tajikistan: Reversing The Tide or The Coming of Age Paradigm?" *The China and Eurasia Forum Quarterly* 6 (3): 101–128.
Logofet, D. 1909. *Na Granitsakh Srednei Azii: Putevye Ocherki*. Vol. III. St. Petersburg: V. Berezovsky.
MSF. 2010. *Turkmenistan's Opaque Health System*. Amsterdam: Medecins Sans Frontieres.
Murray, S., and W. Roscoe, eds. 1997. *Islamic Homosexualities: Culture, History and Literature*. New York: New York University Press.
Olufsen, O. 1911. *The Emir of Bokhara and His Country: Journeys and Studies in Bokhara*. London: William Heinemann.
Oostvogels, R. 2005. "HIV and Men Who Have Sex With Men in Kyrgyz Republic. Assessment and Review." Prepared for Republican AIDS Centre and the GFATM. Bishkek.
Open Society Foundations. 2011. *Pretrial Detention and Health: Unintended Consequences, Deadly Results*. New York: Open Society Foundations.
OSI. 2007. *Access to Health Care for LGBT People in Kyrgyzstan*. Open Society Institute: A Sexual Health and Rights Project/ Soros Foundation–Kyrgyzstan. Bishkek.
Ostroumov, N. 1896. *Sarty. Etnograficheskie Materialy*. Tashkent: Izdanie Knizhnogo Magazina "Bukinist".
Pahlen, K. 1964. *Mission to Turkestan: Being the Memoirs of Count K.K. Pahlen*. London: Oxford University Press.
Peschereva, E. 1927. "Prazdnik Tiul'pana (Lola) v Sel. Isfara Kokandskogo Uezda." In *V. V. Bartol'du: Turkestanskie Druz'ia, Ucheniki i Pochitateli*, edited by A. Shmidt and E. Betger, 374–384. Tashkent: Obschestvo dlia Izucheniia Tadzhikistana i Iranskikh Narodnostei za Ego Predelami.
PSI. 2010. "Kazakhstan, Kyrgyzstan, Tajikistan (2010): HIV and TB TRaC Study Among Men Who Have Sex With Men in Almaty, Bishkek, Chui, and Dushanbe." Round 1. http://www.dialogueproject.org/eng/publications_and_resources/project_publications/research_reports/#go
Renton, A., D. Gzirishvilli, G. Gotsadze, and J. Godinho. 2006. "Epidemics of HIV and Sexually Transmitted Infections in Central Asia: Trends, Drivers and Priorities for Control." *The International Journal of Drug Policy* 17 (6): 494–503.
Republican AIDS Centre. 2010. "Number of HIV-Infected Individuals in The Republic of Tajikistan by October 1, 2010." Unpublished document.
Rhodes, T., M. Simic, S. Baros, L. Platt, and B. Zikic. 2008. "Police Violence and Sexual Risk Among Female and Transvestite Sex Workers in Serbia: Qualitative Study." *BMJ* 337: a811.
Sahadeo, J. 2007. *Russian Colonial Society in Tashkent, 1865–1923*. Bloomington and Indianapolis: Indiana University Press.
Sarang, A., T. Rhodes, N. Sheon, and K. Page. 2010. "Policing Drug Users in Russia: Risk, Fear, and Structural Violence." *Substance Use and Misuse* 45 (6): 813–835.
Schuyler, E. 1966. *Turkistan: Notes of a Journey in Russian Turkistan, Kokand, Bukhara and Kuldja*. London: Routledge and Kegan Paul.
Sidorov, A. 2008. "The Russian Criminal Tattoo: Past and Present." In *Russian Criminal Tattoo Encyclopaedia*, edited by D. Baldaev, S. Vasiliev and A. Sidorov, Vol. III, 16–43. Göttingen: Fuel.
Smolak, A. 2010. "Contextual Factors Influencing HIV Risk Behaviour in Central Asia." *Culture, Health and Sexuality* 12 (5): 515–527.
Thorne, C., N. Ferencic, R. Malyuta, J. Mimica, and T. Niemiec. 2010. "Central Asia: Hotspot in The Worldwide HIV Epidemic." *The Lancet Infectious Diseases* 10 (7): 479–488.
Todd, C., M. Khakimov, G. Giyasova, M. Saad, B. Botros, J. Sanchez, J. Carr, and K. Earhart. 2009. "Prevalence and Factors Associated With Human Immunodeficiency Virus Infection Among Sex Workers in Samarkand, Uzbekistan." *Sexually Transmitted Diseases* 36 (2): 70–72.
Tukeyev, M. 2010. "HIV Infection Epidemiological Situation in The Republic of Kazakhstan."

Tukeyev, M., L. Ganina, A. Yelizarieva, I. Petrenko, T. Balabayev, E. Kudusova, and Zh. Trumova. 2011. *2006–2010 Kazakhstan National AIDS Programme Progress Report*. Almaty.

Universal Periodic Review Submission on Sexual Rights in Tajikistan. 2011. Twelfth Session of the Universal Periodic Review. http://labrys.kg/files/Labrys__Equal_Opportunities__SRI_-_Joint_Submission_-_TAJIKISTAN_-_Oct._2011.pdf

UNOCHA IRIN. 2004. "Tajikistan: Gay Rights Face Uphill Struggle." http://www.irinnews.org/Report/24445/TAJIKISTAN-Gay-rights-face-uphill-struggle

Uzbekistan Multisectoral Expert Council. 2010. "Continuing Scale Up of The Response to HIV in Uzbekistan, With Particular Focus on Most at Risk Populations." Proposal, Rolling Continuation Channel. For more information, see: http://www.undp.uz/en/projects/project.php?id=173

van der Veur, D. 2004. *Kyrgyzstan: "The Country of Human Rights"... But Not For Homosexuals!* Amsterdam: COC Netherlands/HIVOS.

Vereschagin, V. 1900. *Batchi i Opiumoedy*. Moscow: I. N. Kushnerev i Ko.

Vinogradov, V. 2008. *Report on Behavioural Study Among MSM to Assess the Level of HIV/AIDS Risk Behaviour and Factors Impeding Prevention Efforts*. Dushanbe: UNDP.

Wilkinson, C., and A. Kirey. 2010. "What's In a Name? The Personal and Political Meanings of 'LGBT' for Non-Heterosexual and Transgender Youth in Kyrgyzstan." *Central Asian Survey* 29 (4): 485–499.

Wolfe, D., R. Elovich, A. Boltaev, and D. Pulatov. 2008. "HIV in Central Asia: Tajikistan, Uzbekistan and Kyrgyzstan." In *Public Health Aspects of HIV/AIDS in Low and Middle Income Countries*, edited by D. Celentano and C. Beyrer, 557–581. New York: Springer.

Kyrgyzstan: still a regional 'pioneer' in HIV/AIDS or living on its reputation?

Svetlana Ancker[a], Bernd Rechel[a], Martin McKee[a] and Neil Spicer[b]

[a]Department of Health Services Research and Policy, London School of Hygiene & Tropical Medicine, London, UK; [b]Faculty of Public Health and Policy, Department of Global Health and Development, London School of Hygiene & Tropical Medicine, London, UK

As in other countries of Central Asia, HIV infections in Kyrgyzstan have increased steeply in recent years, driven by factors such as the sharing of drug paraphernalia among injecting drug users, sex work and other risky sex behaviours, prison settings and infections acquired in hospitals. In contrast to its neighbours, Kyrgyzstan has long been considered a regional pioneer in its response to the HIV/AIDS epidemic, displaying political will and strong leadership, a timely response, and a multi-sectoral approach to tackle the disease. Yet this progress has become increasingly difficult to sustain in recent years, as it has been undermined by political and social instability, the reorganization of the Country Coordinating Committee to fight HIV/AIDS, Tuberculosis and Malaria, the lack of unified mechanisms for data collection, monitoring and evaluation, a high rate of turnover of senior and mid-level staff, stigma and discrimination faced by those most at risk, and heavy dependence on external donors.

Introduction

Kyrgyzstan, the smallest and, after Tajikistan, second poorest state in Central Asia, has faced many challenges since gaining independence from the Soviet Union in 1991. Beset by political instability, including two revolutions, it has experienced a series of economic crises, widespread poverty, a breakdown of social safety nets and a growth in criminality and corruption. Yet despite these challenges, it was one of the first countries in the former Soviet Union to mount a comprehensive response to the HIV/AIDS epidemic and adopt policies that reflected best international practices in HIV/AIDS prevention and management. As Kyrgyzstan enters its third decade of independence, this article explores the factors that made Kyrgyzstan a regional 'pioneer' in HIV/AIDS policies and whether it has sustained its early achievements.

We first discuss HIV/AIDS trends in the country and examine some of the key behavioural and contextual factors that are responsible for the spread of the disease, including injecting drug use, sex work, sex between men, prison settings, migration, mother-to-child transmission and nosocomial infections (infections acquired in hospitals). The article then explores why Kyrgyzstan has been viewed as a pioneer in HIV prevention and control in Central Asia and among other former Soviet countries. We assess recent HIV/AIDS policies in Kyrgyzstan in the light of common elements of HIV/AIDS policies that were successful in other parts of the world (political will and strong leadership, timely response and a multi-sectoral approach). This is followed by a discussion of current challenges of programme implementation, including the vertical structure of HIV/AIDS programmes, donor dependence and lack of domestic funding, lack of unified mechanisms for data collection and monitoring and evaluation, risky behaviours, such as injecting drug use, and the stigma and discrimination faced by people living with HIV/AIDS.

We conclude that Kyrgyzstan still does much better than many of its neighbours, but that its relative success has been increasingly difficult to sustain. Its HIV/AIDS policy has suffered from the effects of the recent political and social instability, high turnover of senior and mid-level staff, the reorganization of the Country Coordinating Committee, and delays in the allocation of funding from external donors. The strong reliance on external agencies is a particular challenge. Donor efforts, often uncoordinated and overlapping, are likely to face cutbacks in funding in the near future, and undermine national ownership and analytical and decision-making capacity. Yet, without them, current policies would be even more difficult to sustain.

HIV/AIDS trends and causal factors

The first HIV infections in Kyrgyzstan were detected in 1987. Until 1991, registered cases were restricted to overseas students attending a school for pilots (Bashmakova et al. 2003). However, with time, the proportion of new infections among the local population increased and, according to the National AIDS Centre data, by 2001 a total of 149 HIV cases had been registered, including 15 cases among citizens of other countries (Murzalieva et al. 2009).

Since 2001, like other Central Asian countries, Kyrgyzstan has witnessed an increasing incidence of HIV/AIDS, thought to reflect a combination of improved surveillance and a deterioration of the epidemiological situation (CMCC 2010a). In 2009, the number of new HIV cases peaked at 686 (Figure 1) (EuroHIV 2011). As of 1 October 2012, a total of 4469 HIV infections were officially registered in Kyrgyzstan, representing a prevalence of less than 0.1% (CCC 2012b). However, this is likely to be an underestimate: the Joint United Nations Programme on HIV/AIDS (UNAIDS 2011) estimated that around 9800 people are living with HIV/AIDS in

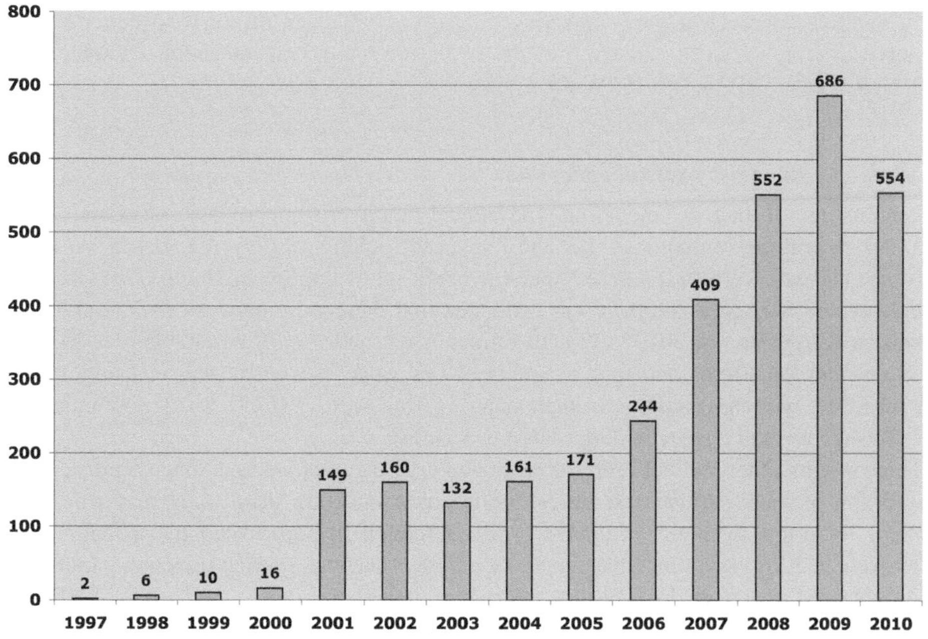

Figure 1. New officially registered HIV infections in Kyrgyzstan by year of diagnosis, 1997–2010. Data sources: Bashmakova et al. 2009; EuroHIV 2011; Ministry of Health 2012.

Kyrgyzstan, while the Ministry of Health (CCC 2012a) puts this figure at 12,040 people. In 2011, injecting drug use accounted for 60.2% of newly registered HIV cases in Kyrgyzstan, while heterosexual transmission continues to increase, accounting for 30.3% of new infections in 2011 (CCC 2012a).

Injecting drug use

Just as Central Asia was once famous for being part of the Silk Road, it is now infamous for being a narcotics transit route from Afghanistan into Russia and then to Europe and beyond (Wolfe et al. 2008). The massive increase in the volume of drug production in Afghanistan has led to a substantial fall in prices, making drugs more affordable to the populations of Central Asian countries (Beyrer et al. 2010; Godinho et al. 2004). Between 1999 and 2003, there was a five-fold increase in the registered number of injecting drug users in Kyrgyzstan, which was followed by a subsequent 20% increase in 2005–8 (CMCC 2010a; Mounier et al. 2007). According to official statistics, there were 10,171 registered drug users in Kyrgyzstan by January 2011, of whom 73.5% were injecting drug users (CCC 2012a). However, once again, international agencies consider this figure an underestimate, and various estimates range from 25,000 to 100,000 drug users (UNODC/EHRN/ECCB 2011).

As mentioned above, injecting drug users remain the group with highest HIV rates (UNODC/EHRN/ECCB 2011). According to sentinel surveillance data, almost 8% of injecting drug users were HIV positive in 2007, increasing to 14.6% in 2010 (Bashmakova et al. 2009; CCC 2012a). In addition to some needle and syringe sharing (in 2011 about 70% reported use of sterile injecting equipment during the last injection), many injecting drug users report hazardous sexual behaviour and irregular condom use, increasing the risk of infecting their partners (CCC 2012a; Mounier et al. 2007). According to sentinel surveillance, in 2011 only half (49.4%) of injecting drug users reported condom use in their last sexual encounter (CCC 2012a). Even though drug use has been decriminalized in Kyrgyzstan, the police forces often take a punitive approach towards injecting drug users, which in turn drives them away from contact with state services and contributes to further risk-taking behaviour (Latypov 2008, 2009; Spicer et al. 2011a, 2011b; Wolfe 2005).

Sex work and other risky sexual behaviours

A combination of factors, including widespread impoverishment, lack of social support, increased mobility, criminal networks and human trafficking all played a part in the increase of commercial sex work in the years since the break-up of the Soviet Union (CEEHRN 2005; Nashkhoev and Sergeyev 2008). It was estimated that there were between 5900 and 8100 sex workers in Kyrgyzstan in 2010, although estimates are necessarily unreliable, due to varying definitions and the stigma and mobile nature of sex work (driven by seasonal migration and high turnover, with new young women entering this sector) (CCC 2012a; Mounier et al. 2007; Nashkhoev and Sergeyev 2008; UNAIDS 2006).

There is some interplay between sex work and drug use: sex workers may spend a considerable portion of their earnings on drugs, while some injecting drug users may offer sex in exchange for drugs (Mounier et al. 2007). Even though it is estimated that about 4–5% of sex workers in Kyrgyzstan inject drugs, risky practices such as sharing injection paraphernalia and unprotected sex under the influence of drugs and alcohol increase the chance of HIV transmission (CMCC 2010a; Mounier et al. 2007; Nashkhoev and Sergeyev 2008). Condom use during sex work depends on many factors, including clients' preferences (with financial incentives not to use one), fear of loss of trust, sex workers' awareness of HIV risks, their ability to negotiate safe sex and marital status (Godinho et al. 2004; Mounier et al. 2007; Nashkhoev and Sergeyev 2008). While in 2009, 92% of sex workers over the age of 25 responding to a survey reported high levels of knowledge about HIV prevention and 94% reported using condoms with their last sexual partner, there has been a decline in the coverage of prevention programmes between 2010 and 2011, from 58.7% to 45.2% (CCC 2012a; CMCC 2010a).

According to sentinel surveillance data, the high turnover of sex workers in Kyrgyzstan may be one of the explanations for their lower HIV-infection incidence (3.5%) compared to other most-at-risk populations (CCC 2012a). It is reported that 25% of sex workers have been in sex work less than a year, while about 20% have been offering sexual services for four years and more (Ministry of Health 2012). However, syphilis rates, which serve as a proxy for risk of HIV transmission, are high among sex workers (26% prevalence in 2009) and in some urban areas, such as Bishkek, they reach 45% (CMCC 2010a).

Sex between men

The latest (2006) estimates of men who have sex with men in Kyrgyzstan range between 18,000 and 36,000, many of whom try to hide their sexual orientation (CCC 2012a). According to UNAIDS (the Joint United Nations Programme on HIV/AIDS) terminology, men who have sex with men are defined as '... any man who has sex with a man, thus accommodating a variety of sexual identities as well as those who do not self-identify as homosexual or "gay"' (Nashkhoev and Sergeyev 2008). Homosexuality was a criminal offence in the Soviet Union and remains highly stigmatized across the region (Rechel 2010a). Although legal prohibitions have been abolished in Kyrgyzstan, men who have sex with men continue to face strongly negative public attitudes and may experience mental and physical abuse (Latypov, Rhodes, and Reynolds 2013; Nashkhoev and Sergeyev 2008).

Men who have sex with men are considered a most-at-risk population not only due to their physical vulnerability arising from unprotected anal sex, but also due to common risky behaviours, such as high numbers of sexual partners, low motivation to use condoms and reluctance to seek and utilize services for sexually transmitted infections or HIV/AIDS (Nashkhoev and Sergeyev 2008; Smolak 2010). Sentinel surveillance shows an increase of HIV rates among men who have sex with men, from 1% in 2006 to 3.5% in 2010 (Ministry of Health 2012).

Even among men who have sex with men who claim to have stable partners, 'casual' sexual contacts are common (Nashkhoev and Sergeyev 2008). In 2008, on average men who have sex with men reported having one steady and four casual sexual partners in the last three months (Ministry of Health 2009). While 86% of surveyed men who have sex with men correctly identified appropriate means of preventing HIV, in practice only 58% used condoms with their steady sexual partner and 54% with a casual partner during their last anal intercourse (Ministry of Health 2009). However, the latest reported data suggests that the percentage of men who have sex with men reporting condom use with their last sexual partner increased to 70.5% in 2010 (CCC 2012a).

Prison settings

Overcrowded prison environments serve as fertile grounds for HIV and other blood-borne infections, which are spreading through injecting drug use and unprotected sexual intercourse. In Kyrgyzstan there are approximately 17,000 prisoners, and, according to sentinel surveillance data, HIV-prevalence rates in the prison population doubled from 3.3% to 7% between 2007 and 2009 (CMCC 2010a; Nashkhoev and Sergeyev 2008). A 2008 study by AIDS Foundation East-West (AFEW) estimated that 19% of prisoners use drugs and 70–80% share drug injection paraphernalia (Ministry of Health 2012; Nashkhoev and Sergeyev 2008).

Continuously high rates of sexually transmitted infections (17% in 2008) testify to the fact that high-risk sexual behaviours are widespread in prisons (CMCC 2010a; Ministry of Health 2009). Since HIV testing in prison settings is still limited (only 31.5% inmates underwent testing and 24% had voluntary counselling and testing in 2008), it is hard to determine what proportion of HIV transmission happens during incarceration (Ministry of Health 2009). According to 2008 sentinel surveillance data collected among 750 prisoners in nine Bishkek and Jalal-Abad prisons, 66% had access to condoms and 79% to clean syringes (Ministry of Health 2009). However, needle exchange and opioid-substitution therapy sites are unevenly distributed among the country's prisons and basic treatment of co-infections and access to antiretroviral treatment are still inadequate (Ancker 2011; Murzalieva et al. 2009).

Migration

The economic crisis following the dissolution of the USSR has led many people from Kyrgyzstan to look for a better life elsewhere. It has been estimated that 300,000–500,000 people migrate every year from Kyrgyzstan to Kazakhstan and Russia for work, mostly on an informal and illegal basis (Reeves 2011; Rios 2006). The funds they remit have become an important part of Kyrgyzstan's economy, accounting for an estimated US$1500 million in 2011 (IOM 2012; Rios 2006).

Although accurate estimates of HIV prevalence in this diverse group are difficult, migration has become one of the factors behind growing HIV rates in the region (Nashkhoev and Sergeyev 2008). Uprooted from their home environments and established social networks, often living and working in dismal conditions, and lonely and alienated in host societies, migrants are more likely to practise risky behaviours, such as alcohol and drug abuse, which may contribute to unprotected sex. This in turn leaves them vulnerable to HIV and other sexually transmitted infections, which can be further transmitted to sexual partners back home and during subsequent periods of migration (Herdt 1997; Smolak 2010; UNAIDS 2002).

Young people

Young people in Kyrgyzstan are particularly vulnerable to HIV infection, due to physical vulnerability, particularly in the case of girls and young women, as well as risky behaviours, often related to the lack of knowledge on the prevention of HIV/AIDS and sexually transmitted infections. Due to widespread cultural conservatism, conversations about sex or reproductive health are taboo, so that most parents avoid this kind of conversation with their children (Colombini, Mayhew, and Rechel 2012; Mounier et al. 2007). A 2009 survey among 3500 young (15–24-year-old) men and women found that only 35% could correctly identify ways of preventing the sexual transmission of HIV and/or rejected common misconceptions about HIV transmission (CMCC 2010a).

Low levels of knowledge about HIV prevention contribute to more risky behaviours, and almost 12% of respondents reported having sexual contacts with more than one partner in the last 12 months (CMCC 2010a). Furthermore, the median age of initiation of drug injection in Kyrgyzstan is 22 years, and, according to a 2006 survey, more than 5% of high-school students have tried drugs (Bashmakova et al. 2009).

Mother-to-child transmission and hospital-acquired (nosocomial) infections

Between 1997 and 2011, a total of 382 pregnant women were registered as HIV-positive and 320 children were born from HIV-positive women, with the HIV status confirmed in 18 children

(CCC 2012a). In 2009, almost 16% of pregnant HIV-positive women received antiretroviral treatment to prevent mother-to-child transmission (CMCC 2010a). Since 2005, the range of institutions offering services to prevent mother-to-child transmission has been expanding and now includes AIDS Centres, Family Medicine Centres and maternity hospitals in different parts of the country (CMCC 2010a).

There have also been several outbreaks of nosocomial HIV infections in southern Kyrgyzstan. Thirty-six children were infected in 2007, 72 in 2008 and 35 in 2009 (CMCC 2010a). In 2010–11, nosocomial infections continued and by January 2012, 207 cases of nosocomial transmission had been registered (CCC 2012a). Fourteen medical professionals were prosecuted for earlier transmission cases, but protests by the children's mothers demanding social justice and state support continue (Ancker 2011; Murzalieva et al., 2009). The nosocomial outbreaks revealed much deeper concerns about the public-health system, such as lack of adequate equipment and supplies, poor infection control and unsafe medical practices and procedures (such as injection and blood drawing), as well as low levels of knowledge among health workers to ensure their own and patients' safety (Bashmakova et al. 2009).

Why is Kyrgyzstan considered a regional pioneer in HIV prevention and control?

Kyrgyzstan has been hailed as a regional pioneer not only for making progress in HIV/AIDS-related legal and health policy areas, but also for setting up effective HIV-prevention programmes that are resisted by many governments of the former Soviet Union, such as needle-exchange programmes in prisons and opioid-substitution therapy (Bashmakova et al. 2009; Thorne et al. 2010; Wolfe et al. 2008). This pioneering role was also seen in the health sector in general, where Kyrgyzstan has been identified as taking a leading role in health reforms compared to other countries of the former Soviet Union, including those in Central Asia (Rechel et al. 2011). The country has undertaken wide-ranging reforms of health-service delivery, financing and governance with the aim of overcoming the extensive, but inefficient, health system inherited from the Soviet period (Ibraimova et al. 2011). What has Kyrgyzstan done differently in respect of HIV/AIDS and what have been the barriers to maintaining this success in the last few years?

There are several well-known international examples of successful HIV/AIDS policy responses, such as Thailand and Brazil (Singhal and Rogers 2003). However, best practices do not replicate old approaches over and over again, but rather adopt innovative strategies tailored to the local context, such as according to the United Nations Development Programme (UNDP)'s 'know your epidemic, know your response' approach (Campbell 2003; Operario et al. 2008). While the specific nature of programmes in each country is likely to differ substantially there are some key common policy elements that are believed to underpin their success. These are: political will and strong leadership; timely response; and a multi-sectoral approach (Barnett and Whiteside 2006; Singhal and Rogers 2003). These criteria can also serve as a useful framework to assess past and present HIV/AIDS policies and efforts in Kyrgyzstan.

Political will and strong leadership

Effective mitigation of the HIV/AIDS epidemic requires not only sustained financial and human resources, but also long-term planning and political commitment to public-health intervention on a scale that has not been seen much previously (DeWaal 2003). Political will, together with strong leadership, is widely seen as key to controlling the HIV/AIDS epidemic effectively (Singhal and Rogers 2003; Spicer et al. 2010). Good leadership involves the ability to mobilize different stakeholders around shared goals and a common vision, having a clear course of action, promoting communication and partnerships across all levels of the political hierarchy and between governments and donor and implementing agencies, proactively identifying problematic areas and seeing solutions, looking after the rights of affected population groups and ensuring transparency and accountability (Collins and Rau 2000; WHO 2004).

Political commitment to tackling HIV/AIDS in Kyrgyzstan has been one of the highest in the region, as noted both by local stakeholders and international experts (Murzalieva et al. 2007). Although political developments in Kyrgyzstan have become more contested and the last few years have been marked by social and political instability, the early political commitment and openness to new ideas by political leaders and governmental officials laid the necessary foundation for HIV/AIDS prevention and control efforts.

Although short of funds, since independence the Kyrgyzstan government showed its willingness to adopt best international practices. As part of its efforts to promote inter-sectoral collaboration and to be able to apply for the Global Fund to Fight AIDS, Tuberculosis and Malaria (Global Fund) grants, it set up an HIV/AIDS Coordinating Committee under the supervision of the Vice Prime Minister (Godinho et al. 2005). This marked a departure from a purely medical to a more social view of HIV/AIDS (Murzalieva et al. 2007). The Vice Prime Minister was supported by the work of a number of strong and charismatic leaders with vision and drive. Such leaders are, according to Hsu (2004), needed for consolidating efforts and forging fruitful partnerships between different parts of society to mount an effective HIV/AIDS response.

Kyrgyzstan adopted legal and policy frameworks that are more humane and closer to international standards than those of its neighbours (Murzalieva et al. 2007). Along with other countries in the region, it has also acceded to a number of international agreements on HIV/AIDS, such as the 2000 Millennium Development Goals, the 2001 United Nations General Assembly Special Session (UNGASS) Declaration of Commitment on HIV/AIDS and the 2004 Dublin Declaration on Partnership to fight HIV/AIDS in Europe and Central Asia; it has also committed to fulfil its obligations with regard to universal access to HIV treatment, prevention, care and support (Bashmakova et al. 2009). Indeed, today's legislation related to HIV and people living with HIV/AIDS in Kyrgyzstan is almost compliant with international guidelines and recommendations, incorporating improved protection of the human rights of most-at-risk populations and the decriminalization of certain activities (CMCC 2010a). For example, Kyrgyzstan revoked the laws prohibiting homosexuality and voluntary adult prostitution in 1997 and 1998 respectively, and in 2007 eased legislation prosecuting drug possession and use, so that HIV-prevention activities among most-at-risk populations could be carried out freely (UNODC/EHRN/ECCB 2011; Wolfe et al. 2008).

While, in general, appropriate laws are in place in Kyrgyzstan, the HIV/AIDS community is concerned about the interpretation of some legal clauses that are insufficiently clear, leaving scope for varying interpretations by different agencies (Murzalieva et al. 2007). For instance, as noted above, the Criminal Code of the Kyrgyz Republic does not prohibit drug use *per se*. But those possessing more than one gram or captured three times within a year commit a criminal offence, which complicates needle exchange and other harm-reduction efforts (Murzalieva et al. 2007; UNODC/EHRN/ECCB 2011). Furthermore, often there are no normative documents or other mechanisms in place to guide and enforce the implementation of these laws at the local level, so that even well-designed laws are not always adequately implemented (Murzalieva et al. 2007).

Timely response

An early response, linked to appropriate and sustainable targets, has been identified as a key means to prevent a generalized HIV/AIDS epidemic (Hsu 2004; Singhal and Rogers 2003).

Creating effective HIV-response mechanisms takes time and the sooner the process begins, the more likely it is to be successful (Hsu 2004). The benefits include a reduction in HIV/AIDS-related morbidity and mortality and a mitigated impact of HIV/AIDS on families, communities, businesses and the public sector (DeWaal 2003). However, the long-term strategic planning required to achieve these goals is often diverted by short-term donors' goals or interests of political elites, especially since the epidemic has taken a long time to fully manifest itself and those most affected rarely have a voice in the political arena (Clark 1994; Hsu 2004).

As soon as the first cases of HIV were registered in 1987, Kyrgyzstan made the potential HIV/AIDS epidemic a priority and was one of the first in the region to put in place appropriate policies and programmes (CMCC 2010b). The first specific policies were discussed in Kyrgyzstan from 1989 onwards (Murzalieva et al. 2007). At that time, HIV/AIDS was seen as a medical problem, so most of the focus was on HIV prevention in medical settings (for example, blood testing and the safety of medical procedures) (Murzalieva et al. 2007). While prevention continued to be at the core of the response to HIV/AIDS, new national policies were adopted in 1996–2000 (Murzalieva et al. 2007). These included the 1996 AIDS Prevention Law, as well as the 'Strategic Plan of National Response to the Epidemic of HIV/AIDS in the Kyrgyz Republic' and the First National Programme on HIV/AIDS Prevention for 1997–2000 (Godinho et al. 2005; Murzalieva et al. 2007). In 1997, Kyrgyzstan was also one of the first countries in the Commonwealth of Independent States (CIS) to set up a multi-sectoral framework for dealing with HIV/AIDS, something considered one of the best international practices (as discussed below) (Bashmakova et al. 2003).

As the HIV/AIDS epidemic took off and its epidemiology began to change, so did the focus of the Second National Programme on HIV/AIDS Prevention for 2001–5. It identified injecting drug users, sex workers and young people as specific target groups (Diamond 2001; Murzalieva et al. 2007). This involved a move away from a focus on universal testing in 1997–2000 towards more targeted testing of most-at-risk populations, while addressing issues of education and behavioural change among most-at-risk populations and young people, harm reduction, legal support and work with law-enforcement agencies, as well as support and inclusion of people living with HIV/AIDS (Godinho et al. 2005). The Third National Programme on HIV/AIDS Prevention for 2006–10 was extended through 2011, while the 2012–16 Fourth National Programme on HIV/AIDS Prevention was approved in February 2012 (CMCC 2010b; Government 2012). Taking into account local priorities and needs, international recommendations and the current state of the HIV epidemic, the Programme set five strategic directions, which are anticipated to be implemented by a variety of state agencies and local institutions, but overall coordination and implementation analysis will be done by the Country Coordinating Committee (CCC 2012a; Ministry of Health 2012).

Timely HIV prevention includes availability and access to services, designed both for the general population and specific most-at-risk groups. For instance, in addition to key prevention measures (such as access to information on sexual health, HIV and sexually transmitted infections, condoms and pre- and post-exposure prophylaxis, and voluntary counselling and testing for all groups), harm-reduction services should be available specifically for injecting drug users (Ancker 2007; Campbell 2003; Gostin 2004). As noted above, Kyrgyzstan was the first Central Asian state to establish needle-exchange points; these were first set up in the cities Bishkek, Tokmok and Osh, and later expanded to 49 points in a number of cities (CCC 2012a; Murzalieva et al. 2009). Furthermore, Kyrgyzstan's penitentiary authorities have introduced harm reduction services in selected prisons, such as needle exchange, opioid-substitution therapy, drug counselling and condom distribution. By 2011, 19 needle-exchange points were functioning in 12 prisons under the HIV/AIDS Prevention in Penitentiaries Programme (Ministry of Health 2012).

In 2002, recognizing the gravity of the problem of drug addiction, Kyrgyzstan was the first country in the CIS to introduce methadone as part of the opioid-substitution therapy, acknowledged internationally as a key means of HIV prevention among injecting drug users due to its effect on drug-injecting behaviour, while several other former Soviet states (such as Russia) still make it illegal (Bashmakova et al. 2009; Latypov 2009; Sarang, Stuikyte, and Bykov 2007). By 2011, 20 opioid-substitution therapy points were functioning in Kyrgyzstan, including three in prisons, and 1013 injecting drug users participated in the opioid-substitution-therapy programme (Ministry of Health 2012).

Kyrgyzstan, in another innovative approach, has, as mentioned above, also removed legal barriers, such as criminal punishment for sex work, drug use and homosexuality, to enable successful prevention work among most-at-risk populations (UNODC/EHRN 2011). It was also the first country in the Eastern European and Central Asian region to develop an educational module on HIV prevention among most-at-risk populations for cadets of the Police Academy of the Ministry of Internal Affairs (UNODC/EHRN 2011).

Multi-sectoral approach

Recognizing that HIV/AIDS is a problem beyond the scope of the health sector, the concept of a 'multi-sectoral' approach was introduced by the UNDP on the international arena at the end of the 1980s (Harman 2009a). It seeks to ensure involvement, cooperation and active participation of stakeholders from various sectors and backgrounds, including state, business and civil society, in HIV/AIDS policy-making and implementation (Campbell 2003; Hsu 2004; Kelly et al. 2006; Singhal and Rogers 2003). It recognized that an issue as complex as HIV/AIDS requires a sophisticated multi-faceted response, taking into account contextual, structural and other factors, and going beyond the competency of Ministries of Health and the public health or biomedical communities (Gostin 2004; Harman 2009b). However, for the multi-sectoral approach to work, HIV/AIDS needs to be high on the political agenda (Slater 2004).

Many countries have promoted multi-sectorality by means of National AIDS Committees, government bodies responsible for the overall oversight of the national AIDS response (Harman 2009a). These seek to establish links between different state agencies and civil society, provide space for open and inclusive discussions, create networks and partnerships, and promote transparency and accountability (Harman 2009a). In 2002, the Global Fund introduced the Country Coordinating Mechanism, not only to improve the coordination of grant applications from the same country, but also to bolster collaboration of the various stakeholders within countries in a formal and structured fashion (Spicer et al. 2011a). The Global Fund requires its recipients to have national strategy frameworks aligned with the UNAIDS' Three Ones principles, introduced in 2004 to improve the coordination of national programmes through an integrated and coordinated HIV/AIDS response framework: one national framework for the response to HIV/AIDS; one coordinating authority with a multi-sectoral approach; and one framework for monitoring and evaluation (Operario et al. 2008).

In Kyrgyzstan, efforts to coordinate HIV/AIDS activities began early – in 1996, when UNDP headed a Thematic Group on HIV/AIDS that included United Nations (UN) agencies, civil society and international organizations (Spicer et al., 2010). By 2005, many thematic coordination committees with similar goals and programmes were functioning (Spicer et al. 2010). As part of the Global Fund grant application process, all these coordinating committees were combined into one Country Multisectoral Coordination Committee to fight HIV/AIDS, Tuberculosis and Malaria, which until recently was chaired by the Vice Prime Minister (now by the Minister of Health) and includes representatives of different state agencies working in the HIV/AIDS field (for example, public health, law enforcement, education, social protection), non-governmental organizations (NGOs) and HIV-service organizations, technical experts and the international community (Ancker 2011; Murzalieva et al. 2007).

More specifically, the main HIV/AIDS stakeholders include: the Parliament; the Government Office; the national, regional and city AIDS centres and various ministries (Ministry of Health, Ministry of Education, Ministry of Defence, Ministry of Interior Affairs, Ministry of Justice, Ministry of Labour and Social Protection, among others); other governmental organizations, such as the State Agency on Religious Affairs, the Government Agency on Drug Control, the Government Committee on Migration and Business, the Secretariat of the National Council on Women, Family and Gender Development, the National Statistics Committee and the State TV and Radio Company – all, to different degrees, are involved in the HIV/AIDS policy and decision-making process (Murzalieva et al. 2007). For instance, the Ministry of Interior Affairs is a partner in the law-enforcement sector, the Ministry of Justice reviews all HIV/AIDS-related legislation, the Ministry of Labour and Social Protection oversees social-benefit packages for people living with HIV/AIDS and their families, while the State Agency on Religious Affairs assists through informing religious leaders how to promote HIV-prevention messages in their communities (Ancker 2011).

While civil society in Kyrgyzstan suffered from repression in the last years of the Akaev regime (1990–2005) and under Bakiev (2005–10), the country is still the most liberal in Central Asia with relative freedom of the press, an active civil society and vibrant contestational politics (Cummings 2012). Once dubbed the 'land of NGOs', Kyrgyzstan is currently home to over 14,000 NGOs, with an estimated 200 NGOs working in the area of HIV/AIDS in 2007 (Murzalieva et al. 2007). The majority are involved in prevention, distribution of information materials, outreach and care-and-support efforts for people living with HIV/AIDS and most-at-risk populations (Murzalieva et al. 2009). From the onset of the epidemic, international organizations, such as the Global Fund, the World Bank, the UNDP, the World Health Organization (WHO), the United Nations Office on Drugs and Crime, the United States Agency for International Development (USAID), the Soros-Kyrgyzstan Foundation and the United Kingdom's Department for International Development (DFID), have played a crucial role in setting up and funding many HIV/AIDS projects (Murzalieva et al. 2007). They are also active players in decision-making processes and many of them are represented in the current Country Coordinating Committee (see below).

In 2007, despite protests by civil society, the Country Multisectoral Coordination Committee was reorganized and merged with the State Emergency Epidemic and Anti-epizootic Commission in an attempt by the government to avoid duplication between the two structures (Murzalieva et al. 2009). With this, HIV/AIDS lost its priority status, as it became one of more than 40 communicable human and animal diseases covered by the reorganized Country Multisectoral Coordination Committee for 'socially significant and dangerous' infectious diseases. The new Country Multisectoral Coordination Committee also became less efficient and active (Murzalieva et al. 2009). Coordination and information sharing between the various stakeholders suffered, as there was a lack of continuity between the old and the new Country Multisectoral Coordination Committee. The monitoring of HIV/AIDS activities was also affected and implementation of projects slowed down.

Noting these negative effects, in 2010 civil society and other HIV/AIDS stakeholders drove the process of restructuring the Country Multisectoral Coordination Committee once again (Ancker 2011; Murzalieva et al. 2009). As of 6 October 2011, there is a new Country Coordinating Committee, now headed by the Minister of Health, that appears to distribute decision-making power equally among state agencies, civil society and international organizations (CCC 2012a; Government Office of the Kyrgyz Republic 2011). However, its mandate is limited to the monitoring and oversight of the grants of the Global Fund and not of other donors (CCC 2012a).

In addition to the Country Coordinating Committee, there are still parallel coordination structures at different levels, including an NGO Steering Group, a UN HIV/AIDS Thematic Group, an Inter-sectoral Steering Group on Health Protection and Social Care in the Penal Enforcement System, and other working groups and donor round-tables (Spicer et al. 2010). While pushing participating members to communicate and collaborate in pursuit of common goals, these coordination structures have been criticized for duplicating efforts and creating structures parallel to already existing ones (Spicer et al. 2010). At the same time, Kyrgyzstan is the only country in Central Asia that has adopted a sector-wide approach in an attempt to achieve better coordination of national agencies and international development partners (Ibraimova et al. 2011).

Current challenges in programme implementation

The sector's vertical structure

HIV/AIDS prevention and treatment efforts in Kyrgyzstan are the responsibility of the health system and its lead institution, the Ministry of Health (Ministry of Health 2012). As in other countries of the former Soviet Union, Kyrgyzstan has created a separate, vertical system of HIV/AIDS services, which are mainly concentrated in AIDS Centres at various levels in the administration and in infectious disease institutions (Mounier et al. 2007).

AIDS Centres are responsible for the procurement of antiretroviral treatment, epidemiological surveillance, HIV diagnostics and data collection and analysis (Ministry of Health 2012). Currently there are nine AIDS Centres and 46 HIV-testing laboratories in Kyrgyzstan (Ministry of Health 2012). The system of AIDS Centres collaborates with 54 other state services in the areas of primary health, tuberculosis (TB) control, drug addiction, sexually transmitted infections prevention and treatment, infectious disease control and blood safety (Bashmakova et al. 2009; Ministry of Health 2012; Thorne et al. 2010). In terms of service provision, public healthcare providers working on HIV/AIDS include Ministry of Health departments at the national and regional level; national, regional and city AIDS Centres; regional and local health facilities; Family Medicine Centres and Family Group Practices; the National Health Promotion Service; and the Sanitation and Epidemiology Service with its regional and local branches (Murzalieva et al. 2007).

However, cross-referrals and coordination between HIV/AIDS service providers and other agencies or providers of health services, such as for TB (the most common co-morbidity of HIV infections), are often lacking and existing connections are not working properly (Murzalieva et al. 2009; Thorne et al. 2010). Strictly defined mandates for different healthcare providers and, until recently, the isolation of the network of AIDS centres from the rest of the health system resulted in few inter-linkages (including information-sharing), duplication of efforts, unequal distribution of government funding, and mistrust between providers of HIV/AIDS services and other healthcare providers (Mounier et al. 2007; Spicer et al. 2010, 2011a). One consequence of these imbalances is that technical capacity and coverage by HIV/AIDS prevention and treatment programmes vary across the country (mostly being concentrated in big cities, such as Bishkek and Osh) and may not be sustainable in the long run (Thorne et al. 2010, 484; UNAIDS 2011).

To address these issues of integration and coordination, there has been an attempt to harmonize efforts across the HIV/AIDS sector and the state-run health system in general. While HIV/AIDS was identified as one of the priority diseases in the National Health Care Reform Programmes 'Manas Taalimi' and 'Den Sooluk', strengthening of the health system was one of the goals in the Round 10 Global Fund grant (GFATM 2011; Ministry of Health 2011).

Meanwhile, USAID's recently launched Quality Health Care Project aims to assist Kyrgyzstan's health system with management, financing and coordination of health services, including for HIV/AIDS (USAID 2012). Currently, there is an on-going effort to integrate various services at different levels working on HIV/AIDS. For example, some of the traditional functions of the AIDS Centres, such as HIV prevention, treatment and care, have been delegated to primary-care institutions (Ministry of Health 2012). Now Family Medicine Centres distribute antiretroviral treatment, while also following up and monitoring their patients with HIV (CCC 2012a).

Donor dependence

Another major concern in Kyrgyzstan has been the lack of adequate domestic funding to back up the declared political commitment in the area of HIV/AIDS (Murzalieva et al. 2007). Kyrgyzstan, being one of the poorest countries in the region, particularly depends on foreign assistance for its HIV/AIDS programmes, with a heavy reliance on the Global Fund (Nashkhoev and Sergeyev 2008). In 2011, US$5.7 million was spent on Kyrgyzstan's response to the HIV/AIDS epidemic, with only about US$1.4 million coming from state sources, and the rest from international donors (CMCC 2012a). The state funds various ministries (such as the Ministry of Health, the Ministry of Justice and the Ministry of the Interior) and specialised state agencies working in the area of HIV/AIDS prevention, treatment and support, such as the network of AIDS Centres, the National Blood Centre, and the National Narcology Centre (CMCC 2010a). Although so far there have been no systematic evaluations on the efficiency of donor aid spending, a recent Global Fund audit revealed serious issues in grant oversight and management on the part of the Principal Recipient, the National AIDS Centre (Bashmakova et al. 2009; GFATM 2012). This in turn has led to the transfer of the role of Principal Recipient to UNDP, major funding delays and interruptions in prevention programmes and service delivery (Ancker 2011; CCC 2012a).

Other international organizations have also played a crucial role in funding many HIV/AIDS projects. Over the years, Kyrgyzstan has received funding from a variety of multilateral and bilateral agencies, including the World Bank, the German Reconstruction Credit Institute (KfW), DFID, the Swedish International Development Cooperation Agency, the Swiss Agency for Development and Cooperation, WHO, USAID, the Soros-Kyrgyzstan Foundation, UNDP, the United Nations Population Fund and the AFEW (Bashmakova et al. 2009; CMCC 2010a). These agencies have not only helped to improve the normative and legislative basis for HIV/AIDS prevention efforts, but also participated in developing and implementing HIV prevention and harm reduction programmes, as well as case-management and clinical protocols for HIV/AIDS and sexually transmitted infections (CMCC 2010a). In some cases, international funding is the only means to cover HIV/AIDS diagnosis, treatment and care, the purchase of medical equipment and supplies, and HIV prevention activities among specific most-at-risk populations (Bashmakova et al. 2009; CCC 2012a).

However, the Global Fund has assumed particular importance among donors. In 2009 alone, over half of international funding for HIV/AIDS came from the Global Fund, which covered antiretroviral treatment supplies, treatment of co-infections, post-exposure prophylaxis and the prevention of mother-to-child transmission (Bashmakova et al. 2009; CMCC 2010a). Kyrgyzstan has successfully applied for and received Round Two (US$17 million in 2004), Round Seven (US$12 million in 2009) and Round Ten funding (US$22.6 million in 2011), which was later consolidated into a Single Stream of Funding (GFATM 2011). This funding was intended to extend prevention, treatment-and-care efforts, such as HIV/AIDS outreach services for three key most-at-risk populations (injecting drug users, sex workers and men who have sex with men), opioid-substitution therapy, prevention of mother-to-child transmission, HIV/AIDS and sexually transmitted infection testing and treatment, voluntary counselling and testing, treatment of co-infections, and antiretroviral treatment for people living with HIV/AIDS (CMCC 2010a; GFATM 2011). The Global Fund also provided funds for creating a supportive environment for policy change and building local capacity to face the challenges of a growing HIV/AIDS epidemic (GFATM 2011). A portion of the current Global Fund grant was also intended to contribute to health system strengthening, through purchasing equipment for management of sexually transmitted infections and blood-testing laboratories, voluntary counselling and testing offices in Family Medicine Centres, and training of relevant health professionals (Murzalieva et al. 2009).

The heavy dependence on international aid means that many HIV/AIDS programmes in Kyrgyzstan are unsustainable in the long term. It also leads to their fragmentation, overlap and weakening of their potential integration into the overall health system; competition and an environment of distrust among NGOs and civil society organizations; and potentially endangers access to essential medical services for people living with HIV/AIDS and most-at-risk populations (CCC 2012a; Murzalieva et al. 2007; Spicer et al. 2011a). The dominant pilot-study and project-based approach, while catering to donors' needs for quick, reportable results, undermines the domestic need for long-term, sustainable HIV/AIDS outcomes. Heavy dependence on international donors also reduces national ownership, governance and capacity (DeWaal 2003; Rechel and Khodjamurodov 2010b). The current slump in international development assistance, following the global economic crisis, has already put severe strains on the ability of the Global Fund to award new grants.

Monitoring and evaluation, surveillance and reporting issues

With so many funding and implementing agencies involved in Kyrgyzstan's response to HIV/AIDS, there is a strong need for a uniform and common system for monitoring and evaluation (Murzalieva et al. 2009). Kyrgyzstan has developed a series of regulatory documents as part of the overall system of monitoring and evaluation for HIV/AIDS, outlining the responsibilities of all parties involved, designating indicators, establishing reporting mechanisms, producing universal guidelines for data collection and processing, as well as providing a methodology for collecting data on prevention programmes and their clients (CCC 2012a; CMCC 2010a). However, approval and implementation of the national monitoring and evaluation system for HIV/AIDS has been delayed due to political instability, continuous changes of decision-makers and the reorganization of the Country Coordinating Committee (CCC 2012a). As of 2011, systematic data collection, which would include reporting by state institutions and NGOs, was still lacking (CCC 2012a).

Without unified data collection mechanisms and a clear set of indicators, each agency has its own system of data collection, and various donors may impose different reporting formats, so that recipients of external funding have to produce reports in multiple formats, resulting in duplication, inefficiency and stress (CCC 2012a; Murzalieva et al. 2009). An analysis of field activities in 2008 demonstrated that implementing agencies used different methods of client registration, as well as different methods for registering activities and assessing their impact (Murzalieva et al. 2009). Another challenge is that many NGOs, funded by international donors, perceive themselves to be independent from reporting to the government structures and their data submission often depends on their relationship with the National AIDS Centre (Ancker 2011; CCC 2012a). Such lack of information sharing and inter-agency coordination often leads to disjointed and duplicated activities, non-comparable data and a waste of funds and efforts (CMCC 2010a; Spicer et al. 2010).

Furthermore, the absence of clearly defined monitoring and evaluation responsibilities or research skills among staff of implementing organizations means that data are often not collected systematically, their quality tends to be poor, and they are mostly oriented towards the requirements of donors, rather than country needs (CCC 2012a; Murzalieva et al. 2009). The Soviet legacy that persists in Central Asian health systems also means that surveillance often exists only for the purpose of enforcing bureaucratic processes and artificially set standards, rather than to inform policy and introduce better practices (Mounier et al. 2007).

For all these reasons, there are great concerns about the validity of HIV/AIDS data, including the size estimates of various population groups and geographic areas covered (Nashkhoev and Sergeyev 2008; Wolfe et al. 2008). Gross differences between official national data and international estimates and lack of systematic HIV testing with good coverage among the general population and most-at-risk populations suggest that actual HIV/AIDS prevalence rates are probably much higher than officially recorded (CCC 2012a; Ministry of Health 2012). Apart from pregnant women, the general population in Kyrgyzstan, which is formally guaranteed voluntary[1] and anonymous HIV testing free of charge at any medical institution, has low rates of testing (Smolak 2010). Among most-at-risk populations, fear of prosecution and stigmatization leads to avoidance of contact with state health agencies, so many do not appear in official data (Ministry of Health 2012).

Stigma and discrimination

As in other parts of Eastern Europe and Central Asia, HIV/AIDS is highly stigmatized in Kyrgyzstan, with attitudes of fear and hostility towards most-at-risk populations and people affected by infection (Bashmakova et al. 2009; Murzalieva et al. 2009; Operario et al. 2008; Rechel 2010a). Since people in many Central Asian communities and societies rely on their daily social networks for survival and overall wellbeing, people living with HIV/AIDS are inclined not to reveal their status to relatives and friends (Smolak 2010). Lack of confidentiality (despite legal guarantees of anonymity) deters many people living with HIV/AIDS from seeking medical help, coming forward for testing, applying for social benefits and enrolling their children into kindergartens and schools (Ancker 2011; Ministry of Health 2012; Parsons 2010).

Most-at-risk populations, such as injecting drug users, sex workers and men who have sex with men, not only face discrimination, but can be denied access to HIV prevention and treatment programmes and harassed by law enforcement representatives (AVERT 2010; Mounier et al. 2007). They are often detained unlawfully, required to pay bribes to avoid prosecution and forced to undergo HIV testing, which should be voluntary and accompanied with pre and post-test counselling (Latypov 2009; Nashkhoev and Sergeyev 2008; Smolak 2010; Spicer et al. 2011a). Policemen have also been reported to pressurize and demand free sexual services from sex workers (Nashkhoev and Sergeyev 2008). Since, as in the rest of Central Asia, corruption is widespread in Kyrgyzstan, disciplinary measures against those who abuse their powers are rare. Furthermore, similar to Tajikistan and Uzbekistan, there have also been 'doctor-police' raids, in which injecting drug users and sex workers were forcibly tested under order of the police, fuelling mistrust of the state system (Wolfe et al. 2008).

Stigma and discrimination can also result in denial of access to education, employment, health services and social welfare (AVERT 2010). Discrimination can also still be found among professionals in the health, education and law enforcement sectors (Ancker 2011; Ministry of Health 2012). Many medical professionals are reluctant to work with HIV-positive patients, as they fear becoming infected. This fear is partly due to lack of education, but sometimes also reflects inadequate safety measures in healthcare settings (AVERT 2010; Spicer et al. 2011a).

The vertical structure of HIV/AIDS services, with their specialized testing and counselling services, contributes to the stigma of HIV-positive patients and people seeking to find out their HIV status (AVERT 2010). Stigma and discrimination towards people living with HIV/AIDS have important implications for HIV monitoring and reporting, as well as political action. They can create a vicious cycle: stigma and discrimination can lead to a lower reported disease burden, and thus to a perceived lower need for political action and greater complacency by governments, which in turn can lead to fewer services being offered to most-at-risk populations and people living with HIV/AIDS (Moore 2004).

Conclusion

For a long time, Kyrgyzstan served as an example of a country in Central Asia that is forward thinking and receptive to new ideas in the field of HIV/AIDS prevention and control. Our analysis of factors that facilitated and impeded progress in the area of HIV/AIDS shows that success is not always easy to maintain. The necessary measures entail more than just human and financial resources; they require major political commitment, sustained efforts and dedication from different stakeholders at various levels of policy making and implementation: government, civil society and the international community, as well as timely reaction to developments and flexibility to address them adequately.

With domestic political and international donor support, Kyrgyzstan has achieved noticeable progress in the last 10–12 years, building a strong policy and legal basis, developing over 20 HIV/AIDS-related programmes and mechanisms to implement them, setting up a functional Country Coordinating Committee, introducing new clinical protocols (for example, for the treatment of sexually transmitted infections), widening access and choice of services for most-at-risk populations and people living with HIV/AIDS, and establishing harm reduction programmes (AVERT 2010; Bashmakova et al. 2009; Thorne et al. 2010). Like other countries with progressive HIV/AIDS policies, Kyrgyzstan's HIV/AIDS prevention activities go beyond distributing information materials and condoms, and focus on the crucial connection between effective response mechanisms and political processes, a dialogue between the government and civil society, and aligning the programmatic and legal basis for HIV/AIDS efforts with international norms.

However, recent developments, such as political and social instability, quick turnover of high and mid-level staff, along with the disruption of the Country Coordinating Committee's activities associated with its reorganization, and delays in Global Fund funding, all had a negative effect on the flow and continuity of HIV/AIDS efforts (Ancker 2011; CCC 2012a; Murzalieva et al. 2009; Spicer et al. 2011b). Furthermore, within the current response mechanism, genuine participation of representatives of most-at-risk populations and people living with HIV/AIDS in decision-making and coordination efforts is still limited, while donor interests, often uncoordinated and overlapping, continue to drive the HIV/AIDS agenda, undermining national ownership and analytical and decision-making capacity (CCC 2012a; Spicer et al. 2011b).

For HIV/AIDS policies and aid investments to be effective in the long term, they need to be part of overall development strategies that are owned by the state and aligned with national (not donor) priorities (DeWaal 2003; Rechel and Khodjamurodov 2010b). Stakeholders and the wider population are more likely to embrace and support nationally driven initiatives than those imposed by international agencies, which often result in a sense of inferiority and powerlessness, and therefore create feelings of resentment and hostility (DeWaal 2003).

Meanwhile, NGOs and community groups avoid open disagreement and criticism of some donor-funded projects (Murzalieva et al. 2009). Competition over limited resources, lack of transparency over funding flows, and mutual distrust between stakeholders also pose a challenge to a multi-sectoral approach and the quality of programmes implemented (Campbell 2003; Harman 2009a; Murzalieva et al. 2009). As this article has illustrated, in view of the many HIV/AIDS organizations and programmes operating in Kyrgyzstan, communication and coordination between agencies in the policy arena remains a challenge (Spicer et al. 2010, 2011b).

Using trial and error, Kyrgyzstan is learning from its past mistakes and the HIV/AIDS sector continues to evolve. Kyrgyzstan's greatest assets are enthusiastic leaders and knowledgeable HIV/AIDS experts in many decision-making positions and structures, such as the Country Coordinating Committee. They share a common vision, understand the immediate and long-term goals and are interested in advancing the issue of HIV/AIDS on the policy arena. While the slowing down of progress in recent years means that it is debatable whether Kyrgyzstan is still a 'pioneer' in the region, many of its policies remain more advanced than those of its neighbours. A country with a vigorous civil society can turn many challenges into opportunities. However, it cannot continue to bask in its former glory. As this article has shown, there are many issues that remain to be resolved, with a reduction of international-development assistance threatening to undermine much of the progress made in the past decade. Epidemiological data indicate that infection rates are still high; for a major change in this epidemiological situation, a variety of structural and social factors need to be addressed.

Note

1. The only population groups required to undergo HIV testing in Kyrgyzstan are blood, plasma, sperm, organ and tissue donors; foreign citizens entering the country for extended periods of time; and medical staff working with blood supplies (CMCC 2010b).

References

Ancker, S. 2007. "HIV/AIDS: Security Threat in Central Asia?" *The China and Eurasia Forum Quarterly* 5 (3): 33–60.

Ancker, S. 2011. *Framing of HIV/AIDS in Policy Arena in Kyrgyzstan*. PhD field research (unpublished). Bishkek.

AVERT. 2010. *HIV and AIDS in Russia, Eastern Europe & Central Asia* [Online]. West Sussex. Accessed August 12, 2010. http://www.avert.org/aids-russia.htm

Barnett, T., and A. Whiteside. 2006. *AIDS in the Twenty-first Century. Disease and Globalization*. New York: Palgrave Macmillan.

Bashmakova, L., G. Kurmanova, A. Kashkarev, and B. Shapiro. 2003. *AIDS in Kyrgyzstan: Five Years of Resistance*. Bishkek: Government of the Kyrgyz Republic, UNDP, UNAIDS.

Bashmakova, L., M. Mamyrov, D. Sorombaeva, and C. Imankulova. 2009. *Overcoming Global Healthcare Problems: National Response to HIV Infection, Tuberculosis and Malaria in the Kyrgyz Republic*. Bishkek: Ministry of Health, Macro International Inc.

Beyrer, C., et al. 2010. "Epidemiologic Links between Drug Use and HIV Epidemics: An International Perspective." *Journal of Acquired Immune Deficiency Syndromes* 55 (Supplement 1): S10–S16.

Campbell, C. 2003. *Letting Them Die: Why HIV/AIDS Prevention Programs Fail*. Bloomington: Indiana University Press.

Central And Eastern European Harm Reduction Network (CEEHRN). 2005. *Sex Work, HIV/AIDS and Human Rights*. Vilnius: CEEHRN.

Clark, C. 1994. *AIDS and the Arrows of Pestilence*. Golden: Fulcrum Publishing.

Collins, J., and B. Rau. 2000. *AIDS in the Context of Development*. Paper #4. Geneva: UNRISD/UNAIDS.

Colombini, M., S. Mayhew, and B. Rechel. 2012. (in press). *Sexual and Reproductive Health Needs and Access to Services for Vulnerable Groups in Eastern Europe and Central Asia*. Geneva: United Nations Population Fund.

Country Coordinating Committee (CCC). 2012a. *UNGASS Country Progress Report – Kyrgyz Republic (January 2010 – December 2011)*. Bishkek: Ministry of Health, Government of the Kyrgyz Republic.

Country Country Coordinating Committee (CCC). 2012b. *Эпидемиологическая ситуация в Кыргызской Республике*. Epidemiologocal situation in the Kyrgyz Republic. [Online]. Accessed November 23, 2012. http://www.aids.gov.kg/ru/

Country Multisectoral Coordinating Committee (CMCC) to Fight HIV/AIDS, Tuberculosis and Malaria under the Government of the Kyrgyz Republic. 2010a. UNGASS Country Progress Report – Kyrgyz Republic (January 2008 – December 2009). Bishkek: Ministry of Health, Government of the Kyrgyz Republic.

Country Multisectoral Coordinating Committee (CMCC) to Fight HIV/AIDS, Tuberculosis and Malaria under the Government of the Kyrgyz Republic. 2010b. *Промежуточная оцена Государственной программы по предупреждению эпидемии ВИЧ/СПИДа и ее социально-экономических последствий в Кыргызской Республике на 2006–2010 годы. Intermediate Evaluation of the National Programme on HIV/AIDS Prevention and Its Socio-Economic Consequences in the Kyrgyz Republic for 2006–2010* [Online]. Accessed October 23, 2010. http://www.aids.gov.kg/ru/?/=programs/state2006-2010

Cummings, S. N. 2012. *Understanding Central Asia. Politics and Contested Transformations*. Milton Park: Routledge.

Dewaal, A. 2003. *The Links Between HIV/AIDS and Democratic Governance in Africa*. Adapted from presentations at Justice Africa, 30 October 2003 and Oslo Governance Centre, 3 November 2003.

Diamond, T. 2001. *Central Asia Hopes UN Meeting on HIV/AIDS Can Provide a Boost to Regional Prevention Efforts*. [Online]. Eurasianet.org. Accessed July 28, 2010. http://www.eurasianet.org/departments/insight/articles/eav062501.shtml

EuroHIV. 2011. *HIV/AIDS Surveillance in Europe 2010*. Stockholm: European Centre for Disease Prevention and Control/WHO Regional Office for Europe.

Global Fund to Fight AIDS, Tuberculosis and Malaria (GFATM). 2011. *Country Grant Portfolio-Kyrgyzstan* [Online]. Geneva. Accessed May 29, 2011. http://portfolio.theglobalfund.org/Country/Index/KGZ?lang=en

Global Fund To Fight AIDS, Tuberculosis And Malaria (GFATM). 2012. Global Fund Grants To The Kyrgyz Republic. Geneva: Office of the General Inspector, GFATM.

Godinho, J., T. Novotny, H. Tadesse, and A. Vinokur. 2004. *HIV/AIDS and Tuberculosis in Central Asia: Country Profiles*. Washington, DC: World Bank.

Godinho, J., et al. 2005. *Reversing the Tide: Priorities for HIV/AIDS Prevention in Central Asia*. Washington, DC: World Bank.

Gostin, L. 2004. *The AIDS Pandemic: Complacency, Injustice, and Unfulfilled Expectations*. Chapel Hill: University of North Carolina Press.

Government Office of the Kyrgyz Republic (Government). 2011. *Постановление Правительства КР и Положение о Страновом координационном комитете по борьбе с ВИЧ/СПИДом, туберкулезом и малярией при Правительстве Кыргызской Республики. Government Decree and Statement on the Country Coordinating Committee to Fight HIV/AIDS, Tuberculosis and Malaria under the Government of the Kyrgyz Republic*. [Online]. Bishkek: Country Coordinating Committee to Fight HIV/AIDS, Tuberculosis and Malaria under the Government of the Kyrgyz Republic. Accessed October 9, 2011. http://www.aids.gov.kg/doc/Decree_Government_CCM_N617_06-10-2011_kg-ru.pdf

Government Office of the Kyrgyz Republic (Government). 2012. Decree of the Government of the Kyrgyz Republic on 'State Programme for Stabilization of HIV Infection in the Kyrgyz Republic for 2012–2016. [Online]. Bishkek. Accessed November 23, 2012. http://www.gov.kg/?p=7522

Harman, S. 2009a. "The Causes, Contours, and Consequences of the Multi-Sectoral Response to HIV/AIDS." In *Governance of HIV/AIDS. Making Participation and Accountability Count*, edited by S. Harman and F. Lisk, 165–79. London: Routledge.

Harman, S. 2009b. "Introduction. Governance of the HIV/AIDS Response: Making Participation and Accountability Count." In *Governance of HIV/AIDS. Making Participation and Accountability Count*, edited by S. Harman and F. Lisk, 1–8. London: Routledge.

Herdt, G. 1997. "Sexual Cultures and Population Movement: Implications for AIDS and STDs." In *Sexual Cultures and Migration in the Era of AIDS. Anthropological and Demographic Perspectives*, edited by G. Herdt, 3–23. New York: Oxford University Press.

Index

Note: Page numbers in **bold** type refer to **figures**
Page numbers in *italic* type refer to *tables*
Page numbers followed by 'n' refer to notes